The Little Book of Child and Adolescent Development

Karen J. Gilmore
AND Pamela Meersand

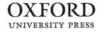

OXFORD
UNIVERSITY PRESS

OXFORD
UNIVERSITY PRESS

Oxford University Press is a department of the University of Oxford.
It furthers the University's objective of excellence in research,
scholarship, and education by publishing worldwide.

Oxford   New York
Auckland   Cape Town   Dar es Salaam   Hong Kong   Karachi
Kuala Lumpur   Madrid   Melbourne   Mexico City   Nairobi
New Delhi   Shanghai   Taipei   Toronto

With offices in
Argentina   Austria   Brazil   Chile   Czech Republic   France   Greece
Guatemala   Hungary   Italy   Japan   Poland   Portugal   Singapore
South Korea   Switzerland   Thailand   Turkey   Ukraine   Vietnam

Oxford is a registered trademark of Oxford University Press
in the UK and certain other countries.

Published in the United States of America by
Oxford University Press
198 Madison Avenue, New York, NY 10016

Library of Congress Cataloging-in-Publication Data
Gilmore, Karen J., 1948– author.
The little book of child and adolescent development / Karen J. Gilmore, Pamela Meersand.
    p. ; cm.
Includes bibliographical references and index.
ISBN 978-0-19-989922-7 (alk. paper)
I. Meersand, Pamela, 1956– author.   II. Title.
[DNLM: 1. Child Development.   2. Child Psychology—methods.   3. Adolescent
Development.   4. Adolescent Psychology—methods.   5. Psychoanalytic Theory. WS 105]
RJ499
618.92'89—dc23
2014019490

This material is not intended to be, and should not be considered, a substitute for medical or other
professional advice. Treatment for the conditions described in this material is highly dependent
on the individual circumstances. And, while this material is designed to offer accurate information
with respect to the subject matter covered and to be current as of the time it was written, research
and knowledge about medical and health issues is constantly evolving and dose schedules for
medications are being revised continually, with new side effects recognized and accounted for
regularly. Readers must therefore always check the product information and clinical procedures
with the most up-to-date published product information and data sheets provided by the
manufacturers and the most recent codes of conduct and safety regulation. The publisher and the
authors make no representations or warranties to readers, express or implied, as to the accuracy or
completeness of this material. Without limiting the foregoing, the publisher and the authors make
no representations or warranties as to the accuracy or efficacy of the drug dosages mentioned in the
material. The authors and the publisher do not accept, and expressly disclaim, any responsibility
for any liability, loss or risk that may be claimed or incurred as a consequence of the use and/or
application of any of the contents of this material.

9 8 7 6 5 4 3 2 1
Printed in the United States of America
on acid-free paper

Contents

Disclosure Statements

There are no conflicts to disclose. I am clinical professor of psychiatry at Columbia University College of Physicians and Surgeons, and training and supervising analyst at the Columbia University Center for Psychoanalytic Training and Research. There are no funding sources or other possible conflicts of interest. Karen Gilmore, M.D.

I have no conflicts to disclose. I am assistant professor of medical psychology in the Department of Psychiatry, Columbia University, and training/supervising analyst and director, Child Division, at Columbia University Center for Psychoanalytic Training and Research. I am associated with no funding sources and there are no possible conflicts of interest. Pamela Meersand, Ph.D.

A Psychoanalytic Orientation to Development in the Twenty-First Century

The Challenge

In attempting to craft a concise introduction to human development, we face a near impossible task in contemporary psychoanalysis. Psychoanalytic theories of development, like their associated psychoanalytic schools, suffer from proliferation, fractionation, and a scarcity of shared theoretical assumptions. Moreover, the lack of empirical foundations (with the exception of attachment theory) and the failure to interface and integrate with progress in other disciplines, such as biological research, neuroscience, and trends in theory-making, has marginalized the entire field (Stepansky, 2009), leaving the many developmental theories embedded within the various schools untouched. Among these, a significant proportion are "part" theories (ibid), tilted toward infancy and early childhood; they produce "psychoanalytic babies" (Thoma & Kachele, 1987; Tolpin, 1989) who (mostly) bear little resemblance to actual babies, who fail to thrive because their schools abandon them after early childhood, and who are rarely nurtured by the fruits of advances in developmental science. In fact, many theories, or at least some of their important adherents, openly discredit attempts to align developmental research and findings with the developmental theories of their school; they dispute the psychoanalytic value of any observational data when obtained outside of the consulting room (Wolff, 1996). In the view of some commentators, efforts to integrate psychoanalytic theories with each other, or to maintain a pluralistic field, and/or keep pace with scientific progression have foundered on the shoals of insular partisanship (Stepansky, 2009). In this book, we sweep aside these differences and the historical resistance to the integration of new scientific knowledge with an admittedly biased broom: We propose a developmental orientation that incorporates what we consider fundamentals of psychoanalytic thinking and developmental science, creating an open system that can be inclusive and reconfigured in pace with knowledge. Developmental thinking is work in progress and subject to continuous correction and augmentation. Although discovery may not find immediate application in psychoanalytic theorizing or clinical work, the active interface between psychoanalytic developmental theories and developmental science keeps our theory-making an organic, evolving process in sync with contemporary society, ultimately enriching psychoanalytic theory and clinical work. And although postmodern theories may disavow interest in childhood history, many were themselves offspring of new findings from developmental research. Indeed, it has been argued that developmental thinking is the premiere fount of creativity in psychoanalysis (Govrin, 2006). We believe that vibrant and relevant psychoanalytic developmental thinking adds a crucial component to twenty-first century developmental science and psychiatry, highlighting the importance of the mind of the child and the autobiographical narratives that shape adult experience: The child is (and always will be) the father to the man (Cooper, 1989; Freud, 1938).

Our Position in the Psychoanalytic Terrain

In brief, the fractionated landscape can be divided, for our purposes, between the *traditional* or classical theories (see glossary) originating before 1980 and the postmodern or post-postmodern schools that have proliferated over the last three decades. Traditional schools—those that emerged before 1980—have detailed developmental ideas that are more or less comprehensive. Most incorporate some version of Freud's original psychosexual progression, but these developmental theories vary considerably in their school-specific notions of psychopathology, their concepts of therapeutic action, and their interest in actually observing infants and children to test their hypotheses. The traditional developmental theories originated in psychoanalytic explorations of the mental life of adults and children, but some have incorporated and integrated observational and research data, depending, of course, on its approach and theoretical bias (Fajardo, 1993, 1998).[1] In contrast, the psychoanalytic schools emerging in the last decades of the twentieth century, the postmodern or post-postmodern schools, which, as noted, have arguably sprung from advances in infant observation, question the clinical utility of developmental thinking and data, childhood history (Govrin, 2006), remembering and reconstruction (Blum, 2003a,b; Fonagy, 2003), and the mind of child. The here-and-now is the primary focus of exploration, and the here-and-now is not mined for its illumination of the past. Even those who utilize observations of mother–infant interactions to clarify the psychoanalytic situation are not truly developmental by our definition, because they do not explore the complex transformational journey from infancy to the adult on the couch. As noted, many contemporary analysts from the gamut of theoretical positions argue persuasively that developmental theory and/or research findings are outside the purview of psychoanalysis (Auchincloss & Vaughan, 2001; Wolff, 1996).

In this context, we position ourselves in the pre-postmodern camp, because we believe in the centrality of emergent ego capacities as a crucial aspect of developmental progression and because we adhere to the idea that effective treatment establishes links to childhood history and facilitates continuous and coherent self-representation. Our orientation is a highly selective amalgam of psychoanalytic ideas and relevant information from general theories of development and empirical research: an integration of ego-psychological psychoanalytic thinking, developmental science, stage thinking, systems theory, intrapsychic and environmental considerations, and one- and two-person psychology. Our utilization of developmental research as a rich source of data and our openness to multiple theoretical approaches to developmental progression is, we believe, in the tradition of Anna Freud's emphatic endorsement of actually *looking at children*, thereby gaining opportunity to see developmental transformations and the synthetic function in action (A Freud, 1963, 1981). Moreover, despite her theoretical conservatism, she offered an early example of *nonlinear systems* thinking (i.e., the integration of complex strands of development in multiple arenas—see glossary) in her proposal of *developmental lines* (Mayes, 1999).[2]

We unapologetically embrace a degree of pluralism that, despite prominent proponents such as Pine (1988), has historically been disparaged among some psychoanalysts as "cut and paste" (Demos, 2001) or model-mixing theories (Mitchell, 1988). According to Stepansky (2009), pluralism in psychoanalysis has begotten only a "plurality of theories" (p. 110). We consider our synthesis to be an integration of these pluralisms so that at the very least, there is a psychoanalytic baby, toddler, latency age child, adolescent, and emerging adult that is recognizable to psychoanalysts at large and yet open to shifts in emphasis, new information, or advances in science. We are heartened by the words of developmental scientist, Alison Gopnik: "being a pluralist does not mean being a wimp. For any particular developmental phenomenon, one theory or another will be true, and we want to know which one it is" (Gopnik, 1996, p. 221). That we freely utilize "theory fragments, almost-theories, and pseudotheories" (Gopnik, 1996, p. 221)—what Stepansky calls "part-theories"—reflects the reality that developmental scientists increasingly acknowledge: "The fact of the matter is we do not yet have a theory of development, and perhaps we never will" (Keller, 2005). There is no unified theory in psychoanalysis or in general psychology. Even the holistic postmodern approach of systems thinking, in ascendance for roughly half a century, has its detractors and, like most new ideas, has been critiqued, defended, and finally diminished in its absolute hegemony, although still profoundly applicable to many phenomena (Berman, 1996; L'Abate & Colondier, 1987; Thelen & Bates, 2003).

However, to the extent that any classical theory presumes to discover the origins of all mental phenomena in mental conflict (as delineated in classical metapsychology [Rapaport & Gill, 1959]) we diverge and decamp. We share the conviction that neurotic psychopathology originates in childhood, that transference contains crucial elements of the patient's past relationships that enter into the co-construction of the here and now, and that therapeutic technique involves transference exploration in order to understand its meaning and gain access to childhood dynamics, positions, and conflicts; however, these propositions do not demonstrate that the "roots and causes" of mental phenomenon can be discovered by the analytic method. The psychoanalytic method examines the historical vicissitudes of object relations, fantasy, cognitive capacities, talents and drives, but cannot say that prodigious musical talent, for example, has a "psychological cause." We nonetheless believe that psychoanalytic exploration of personal history is fundamental to the treatment process, in contrast to "post-postmodern thinkers" who have (more or less) dispensed with the baby in favor of the here-and-now and the equal contributions of patient and analyst to transferences. However, in keeping with the spirit of developmental scientists, insights and new perspectives from contemporary theories "bobbing about around us" (Gopnik, 1996, p. 221) are incorporated into our thinking when they fit the phenomena being considered.

Contemporary Developmental Science

The larger field of developmental science has its own theoretical controversies and its own struggle with causality. Nonlinear systems theory, a paradigm that was applied to psychological entities since its early origins in family work, conceptualizes processes in ways that resonate with psychoanalytic notions of complex, multiply determined transformative exchanges between environment and inner life (Seligman, 2003). Systems theory is especially favored by the co-constructionist post-postmodern schools (Demos, 2001, 2007) because it decenters causality, leading to the characterization of both the psychoanalytic endeavor and human development as transactional processes that self-organize. Dynamic systems theory does away with the Aristotelian notion of "efficient cause;" that is, the assumption that an event is the result of prior events, in favor of "formal cause," which locates causality in the organization or patterns of component systems that arise from their flow and dynamic exchange to produce a "whole." The second half of the twentieth century reverberated with the rise of postmodern systems thinking, which created seismic shifts in the fields of developmental psychology, sociology, history, and evolutionary sciences, to name just a few. But systems theory also has a "shadow side" (Berman, 1996). Most relevant to this discussion is the usual problem of the newest revelatory theory: Systems thinking has become the explanatory tool applied to all natural and man-made phenomena, leading one critic to complain, "if it is everything, it is really nothing. If all phenomena follow the same system principles, we have no basis for understanding anything apart from anything else" (Littlejohn, quoted in Jurich & Myers-Bowman, 1998, p. 83). The idiosyncratic past history of holistic systems and their components, the unique and specific processes that govern different aspects of human existence, the distortions created by convulsive disasters, and primary causality, even in regard to very limited outcomes, are homogenized by a theory that purports to be entirely free of context and specificity in regard to content. The neglect of the part for the whole disallows the contributions from innate or genetic predispositions and leads to considerations of larger and larger systems to effect, permit, or sustain individual transformation. There is no schizophrenia, only a schizophrenogenic family system embedded in a schizophrenogenic society (Jurich & Myers-Bowman, 1998). Causality or, at least, probabilistic causality is inconsistent with such thinking, as is the possibility that knowledge (of the patient) is, at least in part, independent of the knower (Held, 1995). The theory also can be read to downplay the role of conflict in the transformative process; indeed, "the underlying 'hum' as it were, is the karmic notion that conflict is unreal, that there are no accidents in the universe, and that all systems are essentially perfect as they are" (Berman, 1996, p. 44) or, at the very least, moving toward perfection. The theory thus paradoxically lends itself to a kind of "systemic determinism," similar to psychoanalytic "psychic determinism," which neglects external impingements and catastrophes, context, individual constitution, genetic blueprint, and any other forces not intrinsic to the intersystemic dynamic in its backward search for causes.

In our view, the "shadow side" critique is applicable to the relational, two-person turn in psychoanalysis, especially insofar as the theor(ies) deemphasize the role of biological givens, memory, unconscious fantasy, "deficits" (Pine, 1994), and the events and traumas of childhood that are experienced and contained within the individual psyche. Their position challenges the foundational idea that the patient's history is discovered in the transference and undermines notions of therapeutic action based on elucidation of the meaning of transference enactments and memories that bear the imprint of the child's mind (Govrin, 2006; also see Lafarge, 2012). There is no revelation of childhood templates, relationship dynamics, or working models that point to a meaningful piece of the patient's psyche independent of the knower, and therefore intrinsic to the patient's mental life. In defense of developmental thinking and the psychology of the individual mind, Govrin (2006) critiques such "post-postmodern" theorists' reluctance to embrace developmental theory due to "its objectivized universal childhood stages or psychobiological drives that determine or predict later psychological experience and universalist claims about the panhuman content of unconscious fantasies." Govrin asserts that such a disclaimer is "not only denied by their own clinical material, which itself relies on such formulas, but also threatens a deep source of psychoanalytic thinking and creativity grounded in the conviction that we can 'know' something about another human being separate from ourselves" (Govrin, 2006, p. 526 referencing Chodorow, 1999).

Rejection of pluralism and the findings of related sciences would seem contradictory to the complexity and uncertainty that dynamic systems theory embraces. Like developmental scientists Gopnik and Keller, we consider theoretical pluralism to be a legitimate starting point on the way to (perhaps unachievable and even undesirable) integration. Demos, following the tradition of Mitchell (1988), decries cut-and-paste theorizing as an avoidance of the inevitable incompatibility of fundamental principles with findings of contemporary research; in her view traditional schools must give up hallowed ideas like drive and other biologically based motivational systems, including attachment (Demos, 2001, 2008). However, true to Govrin's hypothesis, psychoanalysts who think developmentally and utilize new findings in developmental science to advance, augment, refine, reconfigure, and broaden psychoanalytic ideas, add immeasurably to psychoanalytic thought: Recent examples include Fonagy's "truly developmental" theorizing about sex (Fonagy, 2008); Lafarge's remarkable blending of classical and new thinking in her explication of screen memories (LaFarge, 2012), and Vivona's revelatory use of current research to refute a "nonverbal" period of development, with repercussions in our conceptualization of infants' minds (Vivona, 2012).

Guided Pluralism

Therefore, with the caveats that follow, we find ourselves mostly allied with the traditional (also called "grand" [Govrin, 2006] or "modern" [Chodorow, 2004]) schools, as "modern ego psychologists." According to a comprehensive exegesis by Marcus (1999), modern ego psychology is a pluralistic world unto itself: It offers a "general psychology *describing* all mental function" (p. 867) (note that *describing* is a far more modest claim than "discovering roots and causes"), focuses on ego development and mental structure, diminishes the preeminence of drive and appreciates other motives, integrates object relations, and keeps abreast of advances in cognitive neuroscience and developmental research. Marcus' definition implies that psychoanalytic theory cannot illuminate *psychological origins* of such mental phenomena as autism, heterosexuality, homosexuality, or addiction—that is, it cannot answer *why* questions—but rather examines *how* the ego grapples to synthesize these and myriad other complex outcomes derived from biological and environmental sources. This is not equivalent to systems theorists' rejection of causality, but rather reflects our humble recognition that knowledge of ultimate causes is not only beyond psychoanalytic research, but also beyond the reach of contemporary developmental science.

Modern ego psychology is thus at variance with the early ego psychologists' versions of "general psychology" intended to elucidate the "psychological origin and development" of all psychological phenomena (Rapaport & Gill, 1959). Even though we share an interest in describing how mental structure is formed during infancy and early childhood—building up agencies, processes, and contents, how development proceeds to its completion, how meanings and motives evolve over time, and how childhood conflicts are rewritten and reissued over the course of a life, we do not claim to know "why." Moreover, despite many commentators' refutation of the antiquated notion that psychopathology can be positioned along a developmental continuum, this idea continues to lurk in aspects of our lexicon and should be extinguished (Rinsley, 1985; Vaillant, 1992; Wallerstein, 1994; Westen, 1990, 2002). So, even while agreeing with Freud's basic assumption that a formulation of the mental life of the child is necessary in order to scaffold the search backward for the psychological history of a given symptom or trait, we do not insist that we know or can discover exactly what went awry in development and at what moment, based on adult presentation and recall. Memory, especially screen memories, are rich veins of psychoanalytic exploration and understanding, capturing a complex mixture of veridical perception, experience, naïve cognition, unconscious fantasy (Erreich, 2003), and moments of personal meaning that have lasting impact on autobiographical narratives (Lafarge, 2012), but they do not offer simple causality.

Phases

Most traditional developmental theories, both within psychoanalysis and developmental science, identify universals in developmental acquisitions and tasks and adhere to the progression of development as a maturational program (without necessarily embracing Freud's singular psychosexual motor). Within traditional psychoanalysis, differences accrue in regard to timing, presumptions regarding normative progression, and relative emphases on psychosexuality, object relations, or narcissistic needs. Moreover, as previously noted, the various schools differ about the value of actually looking at children to confirm their hypotheses (Grignon, 2003). The "grand" schools consistently emphasize early childhood and accept the presence of the oedipal period as a watershed, but they differ in terms of how they conceptualize and weight the oedipal versus pre-oedipal period, how they elaborate development across the lifespan, their interest in emerging capacities, and in environmental impingements. In concert with these theories, we continue to see the oedipal period as pivotal, because it marks a developmental shift that introduces remarkable new capacities in symbolic thought, triadic relations, affective range and nuance, mentalization, and creative imagining, reorganizing prior development and reverberating into the future. It encompasses a revolutionary transformation of the mind and a shift in memorial capacity that essentially alters access to prior content (Shapiro, 1977).

In contrast, postmodern theorists tend to dispense with the familiar developmental stages that, beginning with Freud's psychosexual stage progression, have traditionally served to organize psychoanalytic—and in fact, general developmental—thinking (Lyons-Ruth, 1999). Their reasons for doing so are complex and multiple, ranging from their emphasis on systems thinking, which posits unweighted lifespan processes, to their rejection of preset/hardwired stages/singular narratives (Arnett et al., 2011; Chodorow, 1999; Demos, 2008; Harris, 1996; Hendry & Kloep, 2007), to the political climate that challenges the idea of normative pathways that have served to designate variations as healthy, pathological, or disordered (Auchincloss & Vaughan, 2001). These thinkers, in accord with lifespan theorists outside psychoanalysis, view the developmental process as continuous and universal, extending over the entire course of life, with sustained momentum from birth to death. The formulation of psychoanalysis as a developmental process is more or less included in this thinking (for examples illustrating broad application of developmental ideas, see Settlage, Curtis, Lozoff, Silberschatz, & Simburg, 1988; Shane, 1979, 1980). In contrast, developmental ego psychologists in the Anna Freud tradition, like Neubauer (1996, 2001) and Abrams (1990), disagree with the notion that the process of change during psychoanalysis itself is "developmental" and view development as a limited process that ends with the attainment of adulthood. For them, developmental progression is a series of novel mental organizations and emerging capacities due to maturational advances; once the adult form is achieved, other processes assume importance and account for change.

The current literature emanating from general developmental science reflects parallel tension between "stage thinkers" and "process" (or systems) thinkers. Similar to their psychoanalytic brethren, process thinkers see transformation occurring across the lifespan, arising from the "systemic interaction of different resources and challenges, and not simply the passing of time" (Hendry & Kloep, 2011, p. 71). They consider human development to be a continuous self-organizing process inseparable from the surround. Some of the moderate theorists in this group differentiate among processes that impact human development and acknowledge agents outside the patterns produced by interaction: Humans experience *maturational shifts*, such as the universal experience of physical maturation; they experience *normative social shifts* dictated by the particular culture, such as the expectations about academic capacities or age at marriage. Finally, there are *non-normative shifts* determined by individual resources and prior experience (Hendry & Kloep, 2002). To all these thinkers, generalizations about stages of life, even those confirmed by research, are inevitably a reflection of the culture in which they occur. Although the process of transformation is universal, generalizable, and perpetual, the content and reflections upon these processes are context specific.

In contrast, phase theorists contend that "typical" features and challenges meaningfully identify a given stage and a child who belongs there, even while acknowledging the vast variations possible. Phases are partly determined by environmental demand, but are also solidly embedded in biological maturation, which loops back to pace environmental expectation. Certainly, all individuals in a phase are not alike and all psychological arenas in one individual in a phase are not at the same level of development. This idea is fully incorporated in developmental lines (nonlinear and synthetic) thinking (A Freud 1963, 1981). But, like Anna Freud, we find that such groupings serve to organize our thinking and reflect the environmental reality. Most children grapple with bodily transformations, maturation, and environmental demands in roughly the same time period. Cultural expectations, applied to all children in a certain phase within that culture, have an impact on the developmental experience, including on its timing, especially as the child interfaces with extrafamilial society in latency, adolescence, and adulthood.

Unfortunately, thinking in phases has been equated with rigid linear sequences and normative paths, and has rightfully required correction within psychoanalysis. We are confident that a more open-ended and updated psychoanalytic view of development can serve to redress some real errors committed in the name of psychoanalytic developmental theory in the past. We also believe that developmental phases scaffold understanding of the serial mental organizations that characterize the mind of the child as it evolves and allow us to recognize naïve cognitions that emerge in the mental life of adults. Ours is a compromise position that sees developmental phases as a series of new organizations of multiple individually evolving but mutually interactive systems, replete with variability but nonetheless identifiable and implicitly acknowledged by changing environmental demands.

Errors and Correctives

Many problematic psychoanalytic assertions are part of the psychoanalytic positivist past and reflect the arrogant overreach of the then-dominant theory in mental health. However chastened our field may be at present, some of these ideas nonetheless continue in psychoanalytic clinical thinking, specifically in regard to developmental progression (Gilmore, 2008). As suggested earlier, they arose from an inflation of fundamental and cherished psychoanalytic insights, such as psychic determinism and the genetic hypothesis, into a general psychology without due regard for developmental complexity. In brief, these include the following implicit or explicit proposals: (1) that psychodynamics drive development; (2) that specific developmental outcomes are determined by psychic experience in specific developmental epochs; in other words, the continuity of development is mirrored by a continuity of psychopathology (Bradley & Westen, 2005; Westen, 1990); (3) that we can know what constitutes normal and abnormal developmental outcomes and that we can explain outcomes by examination of mental content (Reisner, 2001)[3]; (4) that observations of infants can be directly applied to the patient–analyst relationships (Wolff 1996), thereby discounting the multiple reorganizations and novel capacities introduced by intervening development; and (5) that environmental and cultural influences can always be relegated to a secondary role. Freud's shift from the seduction theory to the role of mental life and conflict in neurosogenesis was itself never a complete abandonment of environmental influence (Gilmore, 2008; Lothane, 2001); he continued to recognize that the environment deeply influences the form, challenges, and crises of developmental progression and called for observational data to augment theory (Freud, 1905, 1915).

The postmodern emphasis on two-person psychology, intersubjectivity, and their developmental implications are correctives to many of these errors, but can lead to the compromise of certain psychoanalytic priorities. New ideas seem to come at the cost of personal history, the dynamic unconscious, sex and aggression, endowment, and ongoing developmental opportunity that can be deleterious or beneficial. For this reason and others discussed earlier, we demur from an absolute embrace of two-person, nonlinear systems thinking, recognizing that both the systems' model and relational theory emerged historically in reaction to positivist and mechanistic views. In their even-handedness, these theories undermine the psychoanalytic emphasis on intrapsychic life and diminish the violent deforming impact of trauma. Moreover, they explicitly eschew the role of constitutional endowment and genetic blueprint, arriving at conclusions that, like early psychoanalytic thinking, fail to recognize the powerful shaping effect of biological givens.

Classical theorists who utilize systems thinking (see Galatzer-Levy, 1995, 2004; Gilmore, 2008; Mayes, 1999, 2001; P. Tyson, 1998, 2002, 2005; Tyson & Tyson, 1990) have offered pluralistic integrations of the co-constructed present and the patient's childhood past. As P. Tyson noted, while endorsing a systems approach:

> ...developmental theory too must be regarded as useful, as our patients come to us with a past that includes a history of unresolved conflicts. An understanding of possible developmental paths might shed some light on understanding the ways in which old patterns of interacting with others, old patterns of resolving conflict, creep gradually into the analytic process despite the opportunities it offers for change. (1998, p. 12)

Thus while observing the dynamics of the here-and-now, we listen for elements woven into mental life from the there-and-then, in addition to other sources known and unknown, such as genetics, in utero events, biological maturation, environmental influences, trauma, and so on. In this, we believe we follow the lead of many scientific disciplines addressing human development; we acknowledge our particular arenas of interest, recognizing that other vantage points focus elsewhere. Nonetheless, we welcome insights and information from these other viewpoints and from related disciplines, because these illuminate the multiple systems at work in the process of development. The course of individual human development can be best understood as the evolving manifestation of a complex dynamic process, provided there is room in that formulation for pre-existing psychopathology, unfolding genetic predispositions, conflict, the dynamic unconscious, biological maturation, and environmental shifts.

Moreover, as will become apparent from what follows, each system that concerns us directly is a composite of many contributing systems, including variables outside our proper domain—such as the timing and emergence of genetic limitations or disorders, cultural demands, the disorders of bodily growth familiar to pediatricians, environmental impingements, or even the appearance of a powerful salutary person at a critical juncture in development. The recruitment of these variables into mental life is inevitable but complex; linear causal formulations, psychic determinism, or the presumption of infinite freedom have no place in this conceptualization. Nonetheless, we believe we can restore a coherent personal history to our patients.

Core Psychoanalytic Priorities

What makes our perspective psychoanalytic? Clearly, there are many psychoanalytic theories, each with their own view of development, and developmental theories (or partial theories) proliferate in every field that addresses psychology, life narratives, childhood, cognition, sexuality, and so on. From our perspective, psychoanalytic developmental theories distinguish themselves by emphasizing the evolution of mental life, the role of adaptation, the unconscious mind, and subjective experience. Like classical or traditional theories, we incorporate the organizing frame of psychic structure derived from, but not ending with, Freud's structural hypothesis (Tyson & Tyson, 1990). Even without that framework, *most* of the following features are consistent with most psychoanalytic theorizing, to the extent that it includes ideas about development:

First is the prioritization of early interpersonal experience (not simply infancy but early dyadic experience); from birth, this is the fundamental paradigm for development and reverberates in most, if not all, important arenas. This interpersonal environment immediately engages with the infant's capacity for relatedness and shapes its potentials (Weil, 1970). Early object relations are preserved in procedural memory and infiltrate all of development.

Second, we consider the reverberations of maturational transformations of body and brain because these drive development forward. Ongoing physical maturation is the organizing premise of developmental neuroscience, developmental cognitive psychology, pediatrics, education, infant research, and many other related fields. From the psychoanalytic point of view, bodily transformation imposes demands on the mind throughout life. This is the case during the entire sweep of childhood and adolescence as the individual grows into the mature form; it is especially pronounced during periods of accelerated growth, such as infancy and early adolescence, in which rapid changes in size and shape are accompanied by the emergence of revolutionary new capabilities. In the developmental context, the body is a fount of impulses and emerging capacities to be managed, self-regulated, and integrated into the self-representation. The corporeal body anchors self-representation and consciousness in somatic experience.

As a corollary, our approach to psychoanalytic developmental theory acknowledges the role of biologically based ego capacities as well as biologically based drives, emerging at variable rates and degrees in the mind. We believe these exist in nascent form at birth as part of the genetic blueprint. However, potentials are affected immediately by interaction with the caregiving environment, are readily recruited into conflict, and can be seriously compromised by intrusions from trauma and other circumstances that overwhelm the ego (Weil, 1970).

In regard to the ego, our interest focuses on the transformations in mental organization as these unfold serially, replacing one another as new capacities come on line, mature, are co-opted to serve new purposes, and/or fade in importance through disuse or natural obsolescence; new organizations, although momentous and noncontinuous, are porous to infiltration or eruption of earlier modes of thinking, feeling, and functioning should circumstances require or reward it. The emergence of capacities and vicissitudes of the drives are biologically determined, but also highly susceptible to psychological and environmental factors. For example, latency is rapidly shrinking in the contemporary world in which digital media, including instinctually provocative messages, are pitched toward the grade school population (Guignard, 2013). Our psychoanalytic developmental theory recognizes all systems; intrapsychic conflict is only one contribution, although it is the one most susceptible to therapeutic work. The clinician's task in assessing ego capacities is multifaceted. Biological substrate is necessarily a component, and deviations in the patient's historical or present functioning can be detected by an informed clinical ear, even while etiology remains unknown. Current conflict and current environmental demands, as well as cultural zeitgeist, affect the emergence and expression of ego capacities and drives, as do the circumstances of the consulting room; the array we see in our offices is not necessarily demonstrative of what is called into play elsewhere. The demands built into the clinical encounter undoubtedly exert a powerful influence on the available repertoire of both patient and analyst.

The clinical task necessarily includes observing the interplay of the conscious and unconscious mind and ebb and flow of the past in the present—or in other words, the variable and variously motivated, conscious and unconscious, access to unconscious fantasy and prior modalities of the mind. Dowling's idea (2004) of a continuously constructed "horizontal" present is useful conceptualization that extends ideas about memory to what he suggests are fluctuations in access, not only to memorialized experience, but to modes of functioning, thoughts, feelings, defenses, attitudes, and ego states: "I can see and feel only from a present vantage point, through the mind and heart of who I am today to a past that has been shaped and reshaped by my past psychology and now is shaped again by my psychology of today" (Dowling, 2004, p. 203). The term *regression* was used historically to represent a linear retreat to earlier positions, an antiquated conceptualization that relies on the outmoded premise of linear progression (Blum, 2011). Dowling's correction explains the emergence of old modalities without resorting to linearity; it also accommodates the reality that the pace and achievements of childhood development are unique and that the rapidity of change makes more evident the use of prior modalities and the interpenetration of levels that are part of everyone's developmental status. For example, a transient loss of a developmental milestone like toilet training, in the context of an obvious stressor like the birth of a sibling, demonstrates regression, but the decompensation of an adult patient on the couch does not (Inderbitzen & Levy, 2000).

As Tuch (1999) and Cooper (1989) point out, even if (postmodern) analysts never offer a reconstruction of childhood experience, they contextualize their patients and their psychopathology in their life story by utilizing their (the analysts') developmental theories, in order to empathically comprehend how they (the patients) came to be the way they are; one might say that analysts' mentalization of patients includes a consideration of what kind of mental organization received a given experience and what subsequent internal or relational "developmental reconstructions" occurred as the patient matured and revised the memory of it. Childhood mental organizations color the nature of perception, registration, and elaboration of experiences and their subjective meanings into memories and fantasies that persist for life. Fundamental aspects of experience are thus shaped by mental organizations that differ from the current one, contributing to the nature of unconscious fantasy (Erreich, 2003) and highly condensed and meaning-laden screen memories that inform essential aspects of self-experience (Lafarge, 2012). Psychoanalysis of these contents depends on the analyst's familiarity with the naïve cognition of childhood that, in combination with wishful thinking, determines the registration of veridical perception (Erreich, 2003). All childhood memories are received by mental organizations that differ from adults', and most memories, with the possible exception of screen memories, are revisited and revised by subsequent mental organizations and sets of wishes. These central mental contents are accessed anew during psychoanalytic treatment, thereby revealing, by virtue of the act and moment of remembering, information about the way the patient has managed self-representation over time.

Although mental contents are unique to the individual psyche, the progression of mental organizations unfolds in a reliable sequence; despite variability, the mental organizations of a toddler or a school-age child share essential features that call upon the analyst's background knowledge derived at least in part from education in development. Familiarity with the sequential hierarchical mental organizations of development can orient psychoanalytic listening, alerting the analyst to the thinking and voices of the past.

A consideration of what environmental demand or situation brought the patient to treatment is orienting and informs the initial approach to the patient; circumstances can invoke adaptive or maladaptive responses, and their specificity illuminates the mind of the patient. This is especially true in childhood, in which the immature individual cannot choose what suits him or her and must perform well at many things in many settings, but it also applies to other life phases as well. Every child clinician is well aware of encounters with a child who seems to be progressing, but not at the pace expected by his or her particular environment or its components (such as educational institutions and peer groups). We return to the ubiquitous role of the environment in the chapters that follow.

Biologically based drives also follow a developmental blueprint that can be shaped by the responses of the human environment and wider culture. Included among these are sexual and aggressive drives, plus the attachment system that ensures the infant's security and heightens the power of nurturing others to deeply influence the expression and emergence of capacities and mental structure. With specific regard to instinctual drives, the capacity to self-regulate, a hugely important system in itself, is established by virtue of internalization of interactions with the caretaker around states and impulses. This capacity is crucial for adaptation.

Adaptation highlights the importance of the larger environment, historically addressed by psychoanalysts only rarely, especially in contrast to current thinking. Since psychoanalysts are themselves a product of their culture and the zeitgeist of the day, it is a challenge indeed to step "outside" in order to recognize its repercussions in self-representation, self-experience, mental structure, and multiple features of personality development, including new phases such as emerging adulthood. Although the native purview of the analyst is the individual mind, awareness of cultural pressures and opportunities facilitates the process of contextualization. Without comprehension of cultural and social factors, we risk obsolescence in times of dramatic social change that transform fundamental human experience.

Many psychoanalysts from a range of schools have an interest in *mental structure*, which itself emerges from transactions among all developing systems. Even within the relational movement, there is growing willingness to recognize consistency in personality despite the collaborative co-construction that characterizes the analytic dyad. We maintain our interest in structural aspects of superego formation, defenses, the unconscious mind, and the ego, broadly defined. However unfortunate its reification has been and however fluid it may be, mental structure, for us, is a powerful organizing concept provided it is applied flexibly.

Finally, our proposal for a psychoanalytic approach to development fosters the creative interface with the information obtained from other neighboring developmental sciences, because these can provide new insights and clarifications about the processes that concern us (Gilmore, 2008). It seems self-evident that new discoveries in neuroscience, cognitive neurodevelopment, infant research, and so on are of interest and importance to our theory-making, just as awareness of literature and contemporary culture are crucial for clinical sensitivity.

Our Method and Goals

It is not our intention to compare theories in depth, nor do we hope to reconcile conflicting propositions about development that are central to the different psychoanalytic schools. Following Gopnick's lead, we selectively borrow ideas that appear heuristically and clinically relevant and that fit the data under consideration. We organize our thinking about development by phases, because we believe that maturation unfolds in a globally predictable sequence and that the environment identifies, evaluates, and impinges on children based on their capacity to meet culture-specific phase expectations.

We see the developmental process as a vastly complex, nonlinear, dynamic system; nonetheless, in considering any facet or period of development, we highlight components that are especially salient and include history, context, and content. Our goals in this volume are to illuminate the developmental process as a narrative that unfolds over the first three decades of life; to alert the clinician to the penetration of the patient's inner life, unconscious fantasy, and naïve cognitions into the therapeutic relationship; and to sensitize the analytical ear to how the present and past mutually inform and illuminate each other, how the here-and-now resonates with the there-and-then, and how prior modalities of experience infiltrate the transference. Finally we believe that the judicious reading of theoretical advances and the extraordinary discoveries of related sciences and research can be integrated and adapted for psychoanalytic purposes. A comprehensive, humanistic psychoanalytic understanding of mental life cannot be based on arcane and antiquated notions of how the mind develops and cannot neglect the powerful social transformations that affect our practice and alter our patients' mental structure, expectations from treatment, orientation to time, and tolerance of depth.

Our conviction is that a pluralistic developmental framework helps in the arduous work of analysis with patients, both children and adults. Most psychoanalysts rely on the mutual illumination of the past and the present, since, put simply (and admittedly somewhat simplistically) the past constrains the present and the present predicts the past (Hartmann & Kris, 1945); our skill in establishing continuity of the autobiographical self and the integration of past experience depends on our implicit developmental theories. An education in human development and phase-specific conflicts, combined with sensitivity to contemporary cultural demands, provides shape and coherence to the emerging picture of the patient's inner life and contributes to the depth and sensitivity of clinical work.

- Development is a complex process shaped by biological givens, emerging ego capacities, environment, and prior experience resulting in sequential mental organizations that are discontinuous, infinitely variable, but recognizable as representative of a developmental epoch.

• Despite current arguments against developmental phases, they continue to serve as shorthand to meaningfully orient the clinician to probable mental capacities and organization and environmental expectations. Subjective experience can be deeply affected by how good a fit the individual makes with specific features and requirements of the environment.

• Pluralism is the lot of developmental theorists, because no one theory can encompass the range of interfacing variables and the nature of their interactions.

• Developmental knowledge enhances our understanding of adult mental health and psychopathology.

Notes

1. Anna Freud, the pioneer of infant and child observation, was arguably the impetus for the psychoanalytic infancy research movement that burgeoned in the United States (Grignon 2003), but infancy and child researchers who challenged classical Freudian principles, like Bowlby and Mahler, were initially marginalized by the psychoanalytic establishment (Coates, 2004).

2. Her idea of developmental lines is decidedly not linear, despite its terminology: It traces the evolution of potentially synchronous or uneven development in multiple domains that cohere into the progressive iterations of one aspect of personality, such as "dependency to emotional self-reliance," against the "background of developmental norms" (1963, pp. 245–247). Developmental norms are, of course, reflections of environmental expectations and demands based on age and stage. Upon examination, hers is a complex perspective that gives weight to the significance of stages, environment, lifespan evolution, and complex nonlinear systems in the developmental process.

3. Examples of this error are legion in the history of psychoanalysis, including theories about the psychodynamic origins of autism, schizophrenia (Willick, 1990), psychosomatic disorders, borderline personality, learning disabilities, homosexuality (Auchincloss & Vaughan,

2001), infertility (Zalusky, 2000), and the nature of female development in general.

References

Abrams, S. (1990). The psychoanalytic process: the developmental and the integrative. *Psychoanalytic Quarterly, 59*, 650–677.

Arnett, J. J., Kloep, M., Hendry, L. B., & Tanner, J. L. (2011). *Debating emerging adulthood: stage or process.* New York: Oxford University Press.

Auchincloss, E. L. & Vaughan, S. C. (2001). Psychoanalysis and homosexuality. *Journal of the American Psychoanalytic Association, 49*, 1157–1186.

Berman, M. (1996). The shadow side of systems theory. *Journal of Humanistic Psychology, 36*, 28–54.

Blum, H. P. (2011). Introduction. *The Psychoanalytic Review, 98*, 613–632.

Blum, H. P. (2003a). Repression, transference and reconstruction. *International Journal of Psycho-Analysis, 84*, 497–503.

Blum, H. P. (2003b). Response to Peter Fonagy. *International Journal of Psychoanalysis, 84*, 509–513.

Bradley, R. & Westen, D. (2005). The psychodynamics of borderline personality disorder: a view from developmental psychopathology. *Development and Psychopathology, 17*, 927–957.

Chodorow, N. J. (1999). Commentaries. *Journal of the American Psychoanalytic Association, 47*, 365–370.

Chodorow, N. J. (2004). The American independent tradition: Loewald, Erikson, and the (possible) rise of intersubjective ego psychology. *Psychoanalytic Dialogues, 14*, 207–232.

Coates, S. W. (2004). John Bowlby and Margaret S Mahler: their lives and theories. *Journal of the American Psychoanalytic Association, 52*, 571–601.

Cooper, A. (1989). Infant research and adult psychoanalysis. In S. Dowling & A. Rothstein (Eds.), *The Significance of Infant Observational Research for Clinical Work with Children, Adolescents, and Adults* (pp. 79–89). Workshop Series of the American Psychoanalytic Association Monograph 5. Madison, CT: International Universities Press.

Demos, E. V. (2001). Psychoanalysis and the human sciences: the limitations of cut-and-paste theorizing. *American Imago, 58,* 649–684.

Demos, E. V. (2008). Basic human priorities reconsidered. *Annual of Psychoanalysis, 36,* 246–265.

Dowling, S. (2004). A reconsideration of the concept of regression. *Psychoanalytic Study of the Child, 58,* 191–210.

Erreich, A. (2003). A modest proposal: (re)defining unconscious fantasy. *Psychoanalytic Quarterly, 72,* 541–574.

Fajardo, B. (1993). Conditions for the relevance of infant research to clinical psychoanalysis. *International Journal of Psycho-Analysis, 74,* 975–991.

Fajardo, B. (1998). A new view of developmental research for psychoanalysts. *Journal of the American Psychoanalytic Association, 46,* 185–207.

Fonagy, P. (2003). Rejoinder to Harold Blum. *International Journal of Psychoanalysis, 84,* 503–509.

Fonagy, P. (2008). A genuinely developmental theory of sexual enjoyment and its implications for psychoanalytic technique. *Journal of the American Psychoanalytic Association, 56,* 11–36.

Freud, A. (1963). The concept of developmental lines. *Psychoanalytic Study of the Child, 18,* 245–265.

Freud, A. (1981). The concept of developmental lines—their diagnostic significance. *Psychoanalytic Study of the Child, 36,* 129–136.

Freud, S. (1905). Three essays on the theory of sexuality. In J. Strachey (Ed. & Trans.), *The Standard Edition of the Complete Works of Sigmund Freud* (Vol. 7, pp. 130–243). London: Hogarth Press. (Original work published 1916–1917)

Freud, S. (1915). Instincts and their vicissitudes. In J. Strachey (Ed. & Trans.), *The Standard Edition of the Complete Works of Sigmund Freud* (Vol. 24, pp. 109–140). London: Hogarth Press. (Original work published 1916–1917)

Freud, S. (1938). An outline of psychoanalysis. In J. Strachey (Ed. & Trans.), *The Standard Edition of the Complete Psychological Works of Sigmund Freud* (Vol. 23, pp. 139–208). London: Hogarth Press, 1962.

Galatzer-Levy, R. M. (1995). Psychoanalysis and dynamical systems theory: prediction and self similarity. *Journal of the American Psychoanalytic Association, 43,* 1085–1113.

Galatzer-Levy, R. M. (2004). Chaotic possibilities. *International Journal of Psychoanalysis, 85,* 419–441.

Gilmore, K. (2008). Psychoanalytic developmental theory: a contemporary reconsideration. *Journal of the American Psychoanalytic Association*, 56, 885–907.

Gopnik, A. (1996). The post-Piaget era. *Psychological Science*, 7, 221–225.

Govrin, A. (2006). The dilemma of contemporary psychoanalysis: toward a "knowing" post post-modernism. *Journal of the American Psychoanalytic Association*, 54, 507–535.

Grignon, M. (2003). Infant observation: its relevance in teaching psychoanalysis and psychotherapy. *Canadian Journal of Psychoanalysis*, 11, 421–433.

Guignard, F. (2013). Psychic development in a virtual world. In A. Lemma & L. Caparrotta (Eds.) *Psychoanalysis in the Technoculture Era* (pp. 62–74). London: Routledge Press.

Harris, A. (1996). The conceptual power of multiplicity. *Contemporary Psychoanalysis*, 32, 537–552.

Hartmann, H. & Kris, E. (1945). The genetic approach in psychoanalysis. *Psychoanalytic Study of the Child*, 1, 11–30.

Held, B. (1995). *Back to Reality: A Critique of Postmodern Theory in Psychotherapy*. New York: Norton.

Hendry, L. B. & Kloep, M. (2002). *Lifespan Development: Resources, Challenges and Risks*. London: Thompson Press.

Hendry, L. B. & Kloep, M. (2007). Conceptualizing emerging adulthood: inspecting the emperor's new clothes? *Child Development Perspectives*, 1, 74–79.

Hendry, L. B. & Kloep, M. (2011). Lifestyles in emerging adulthood: who needs stages anyway? In J. J. Arnett, M. Kloep, L. B. Hendry, & J. L. Tanner (Eds.), *Debating Emerging Adulthood: Stage or Process?* (pp. 77–106). New York: Oxford University Press.

Inderbitzen, L. & Levy, S. (2000). Regression and psychoanalytic technique: the concretization of a concept. *Psychoanalytic Quarterly*, 69, 195–223.

Jurich, J. A. & Myers-Bowman, K. S. (1998). Systems theory and its applications to research on human sexuality. *The Journal of Sex Research*, 35, 72–87.

Keller, E. F. (2005). DDS: Dynamics of developmental systems. *Biology and Philosophy*, 20, 409–416.

L'Abate, L. & Colondier, G. (1987). The emperor has no clothes! Long live the emperor! A critique of family systems thinking and a reductionistic proposal. *The American Journal of Family Therapy*, 15, 19–33.

LaFarge, L. (2012). The screen memory and the act of remembering. *International Journal of Psychoanalysis, 93,* 1249–1265.

Lothane, Z. (2001). Freud's alleged repudiation of the seduction theory revisited: facts and fallacies. *Psychoanalytic Review, 88,* 673–723.

Lyons-Ruth, K. (1999). The two-person unconscious: intersubjective dialogue, enactive relational representation, and the emergence of new forms of relational organization. *Psychoanalytic Inquiry, 19,* 576–617.

Marcus, E. R. (1999). Modern ego psychology. *Journal of the American Psychoanalytic Association, 47,* 843–871.

Mayes, L. C. (1999). Clocks, engines, and quarks—love, dreams, and genes: what makes development happen? *Psychoanalytic Study of the Child, 54,* 169–192.

Mayes, L. C. (2001). The twin poles of order and chaos. *Psychoanalytic Study of the Child, 56,* 137–170.

Mitchell, S. (1988). *Relational Concepts in Psychoanalysis: An Integration.* Cambridge, MA: Harvard University.

Neubauer, P. B. (1996). Current issues in psychoanalytic child development. *Psychoanalytic Study of the Child, 51,* 35–45.

Neubauer, P. B. (2001). Emerging issues: some observations about changes in technique in child analysis. *Psychoanalytic Study of the Child, 56,* 16–26.

Pine, F. (1988). The four psychologies of psychoanalysis and their place in clinical work. *Journal of the American Psychoanalytic Association, 36,* 571–596.

Pine, F. (1994). Some impressions regarding conflict, defect, and deficit. *Psychoanalytic Study of the Child, 49,* 222–240.

Rapaport, D. & Gill, M. M. (1959). The points of view and assumptions of metapsychology. *International Journal of Psycho-analysis, 40,* 153–162.

Reisner, S. (2001). Freud and developmental theory: a 21st-century look at the origin myth of psychoanalysis. *Studies in Gender and Sexuality, 2,* 97–128.

Rinsley, D. B. (1985). Notes on the pathogenesis and nosology of borderline and narcissistic personality disorders. *Journal of the American Academy of Psychoanalysis, 13,* 17–328.

Seligman, S. (2003). The developmental perspective in relational psychoanalysis. *Contemporary Psychoanalysis, 39,* 477–508.

Settlage, C. F, Curtis, J., Lozoff, M., Silberschatz, G., & Simburg, E. J. (1988). Conceptualizing adult development. *Journal of the American Psychoanalytic Association, 36,* 347–369.

Shane, M. (1979). The developmental approach to "working through" in the analytic process. *International Journal of Psychoanalysis, 60,* 375–382.

Shane, M. (1980). Countertransference and the developmental orientation and approach. *Psychoanalysis and Contemporary Thought, 3,* 195–212.

Shapiro, T. (1977). Oedipal distortions in severe character pathologies developmental and theoretical considerations. *Psychoanalytic Quarterly, 46,* 559–579.

Stepansky, P. (2009). *Psychoanalysis at the Margins.* New York: Other Press.

Thelen, E. & Bates, E. (2003). Connectionism and dynamic systems: are they really different? *Developmental Science, 6,* 378–391.

Thoma, H. & Kachele, J. (1987). *Psychoanalytic Practice: Principles.* Berlin: Springer-Verlag.

Tolpin, M. N. (1989). A prospective constructionist view of development. *Annual of Psychoanalysis, 17,* 308–316.

Tuch, R. H. (1999). The construction, reconstruction, and deconstruction of memory in the light of social cognition. *Journal of the American Psychoanalytic Association, 47,* 153–186.

Tyson, P. (1998). Developmental theory and the post-modern analyst. *Journal of the American Psychoanalytic Association, 46,* 9–15.

Tyson, P. (2002). The challenges of psychoanalytic developmental theory. *Journal of the American Psychoanalytic Association, 50,* 19–52.

Tyson, P. (2005). Affects, agency, and self-regulation: complexity theory in the treatment of children with anxiety and disruptive behavior disorders. *Journal of the American Psychoanalytic Association, 53,* 159–188.

Tyson, P. & Tyson, R. (1990). *Psychoanalytic Theories of Development: An Integration.* New Haven, CT: Yale University.

Vaillant, G. E. (1992). The historical origins and future potential of Sigmund Freud's concept of the mechanisms of defence. *International Review of Psychoanalysis, 19,* 35–50.

Vivona, J. (2012). Is there a nonverbal period of development? *Journal of the American Psychoanalytic Association, 60,* 231–265.

Wallerstein, R. S. (1994). Borderline disorders: report on the 4th IPA Research Conference. *International Journal of Psychoanalysis, 75,* 763–774.

Weil, A. (1970). The basic core. *Psychoanalytic Study of the Child, 25,* 442–460.

Westen, D. (1990). Towards a revised theory of borderline object relations: contributions of empirical research. *International Journal of Psychoanalysis, 71*, 661–693.

Westen, D. (2002). The language of psychoanalytic discourse. *Psychoanalytic Dialogues, 12*, 857–898.

Willick, M. S. (1990). Psychoanalytic concepts of the etiology of severe mental illness. *Journal of the American Psychoanalytic Association, 38*, 1049–1081.

Wolff, P. (1996). The irrelevance of infant observations for psychoanalysis. *Journal of the American Psychoanalytic Association, 44*, 369–392.

Zalusky, S. (2000). Infertility in the age of technology. *Journal of the American Psychoanalytic Association, 48*, 1542–1562.

2

Infancy: Psychoanalytic Theory, Developmental Research, and the Mother–Child Dyad in the First Year of Life

Overview

The first year of life is beautifully captured in the metaphor of the infant's "psychological birth" (Mahler, Pine, & Bergman, 1975), reflecting the gradual formation of psychic structure, the unfolding of the child's unique individuality, and the dawning awareness of the self within the mother–child dyad. While a generation of infant research has reshaped the theoretical landscape, Winnicott's (1975) often-quoted assertion, "there is no such thing as a baby" (p. 99) without a mother, remains a cornerstone of early development: Contemporary studies confirm the enduring impact of the mother's affective mirroring and responsiveness on the baby's emerging brain-based self-regulatory systems and early relational patterns (Balbernie, 2001; Fonagy & Target, 2002; Shore, 1999).

We join a multitude of psychoanalysts in our fascination with the findings of empirical infant research, particularly its elucidation of truly remarkable innate capacities for social-emotional attunement and reciprocity. At the same time, we are indebted to psychoanalytic baby-watchers (e.g., Winnicott, Mahler), whose observations not only presage current thinking about the young child's emerging ego capacities, identity, and sense of self, but are contextualized within rich and complex analytic theories. This chapter provides what is inevitably a curtailed review of a vast body of observational and empirical work, emphasizing areas of interpenetration between psychoanalytic thinking and research in order to attempt a contemporary depiction of the infant year.

Theories of Infancy

Efforts to integrate infant observation with psychoanalytic principles date back to the inception of psychoanalysis (e.g., Hug-Hellmuth, 1919); baby-watching was strongly endorsed at the Hampstead Nurseries and at Tavistock (Bick, 1964; A. Freud, 1953; Midgley, 2007). Spitz, Mahler, and Winnicott are among the prominent theorists whose observations of the mother–infant relationship, and of the "real" mother's essential role in the child's developmental outcome, were gradually incorporated into mainstream psychoanalytic thought (as a sample of their work, see Mahler, 1963; Spitz, 1946; Winnicott, 1956). Mahler's investigations into the dyadic process of separation–individuation, and Olesker's studies on early gender behavior are examples of systematic, observational research that is guided by and further enriches analytic theory (Harpaz-Rotem & Bergman, 2006; Olesker, 1990). However, there is no doubt that contemporary integrations of empirical, attachment-based research and psychoanalytic theory (e.g., Fonagy, 2001; Slade & Cohen, 1996) have fueled an unprecedented psychoanalytic interest in early mental development, with particular emphasis on the processes of mother–infant inter-subjectivity; indeed, a number of psychoanalysts have explicitly linked their own theories to attachment-based findings, with one asserting that such research is "of the highest importance" for our field (e.g., Sandler, 2003, p. 26).

Nonetheless, psychoanalytic thinkers and developmentalists have often found themselves at odds: An historic London conference in 2000, wherein Andre Green and Daniel Stern famously debated the inherent value of infant research for the field of psychoanalysis, revealed seemingly irreconcilable positions (Ackerman, 2010). Andre Green's (2000) assertion that "the findings of researchers look very meager" (p. 21) when compared with the richness of analytic material reflects his conviction that the individual's past is meaningfully apprehended only through the distortions and projections of analytic reconstruction; in contrast, Stern (2000) elevates the role of the infant's immediate, reality-based "raw experience-as-it-is-lived" (p. 82), and points to empirical evidence for its enduring influence in lifelong relational patterns.

Perhaps in milder form, such divisions persist within the psychoanalytic community. The emphasis on behaviorally defined categories and the diminishment or sheer absence of conflict, sexuality, aggression and unconscious fantasy in the attachment research literature, have led many psychoanalysts toward a dubious attitude vis-à-vis the value of empirical studies. Although Bowlby, trained as a psychoanalyst, incorporates notions of defense and unconscious process into his theory of the mother–infant bond, his somewhat static cognitive schemas of relationships, known as "internal working models" are a centerpiece of attachment theory; these remain problematic in the minds of many psychoanalytic clinicians and theorists, who see their main tasks as grappling with the most complex and subtle aspects of individual subjectivity (Fonagy & Target, 2007). Moreover, the inevitable tendency of research to privilege experimental findings that are gleaned during infants' transitory periods of alert inactivity strikes some psychoanalysts as problematic, as this leads to omission of essential, pervasive but less measurable aspects of infant–mother experience, such as states of distress (Shuttleworth, 1989).

However, as the dominant paradigm in contemporary developmental research, attachment theory has exerted enormous influence in academic and more broadly cultural thinking about early mental life. Bowlby's (1958, 1969, 1973) seminal contributions include the premise of a biologically based need for secure attachment and a clear assertion of the impact of maternal day-to-day care; he conceived of attachment as a behavioral system geared to elicit the mother's responsiveness and maintain her proximity, thereby increasing the child's chances for survival. Perhaps most importantly, he definitively linked early disruptions in mothering to later developmental disturbance. The burgeoning fund of attachment-guided research and the ensuing refinement of notions about such processes as mother–infant affective sharing have led to re-examination and revision of original analytic concepts; within the relational school of psychoanalytic thought, attachment findings have been particularly instrumental in building and modifying theories (Beebe, Knoblauch, & Rustin, 2003; Lyons-Ruth, 1999).

We offer just a few examples of interdisciplinary collaboration and cross-fertilization, some of which are explored in greater detail later in this chapter. Areas in which empirical evidence appears to support and enrich existing psychoanalytic concepts include: delineations of maternal mirroring functions, such as marked affect and contingent responsiveness; hypothesized pathways for the intergenerational transmission of maternal fantasies, distortions, and unresolved conflicts, which are shown to involve the mother's reflective and mentalizing capacities; and elaborations of emotional communication and mutual regulation within the mother–infant dyadic system in later infancy, such as the processes of joint attention and social referencing (Gergely, 2000; Stern, 1985). Revision and rejection of long-held psychoanalytic assumptions include notions of the neonate's stimulus barrier and objectless or autistic-like states (Freud, 1914; Mahler, Pine, & Bergman, 1975); these are largely replaced by contemporary theories of the newborn mind as an open system, prewired for social interaction and equipped to discern meaning from the social environment (Bornstein et al., 2006).

More complex notions, not readily available for definitive scrutiny and confirmation, include the nature (or existence) of early fantasy and the infant's subjective sense of merger or separateness. Empirical work largely discounts the idea of ubiquitous unconscious fantasy (e.g., as proposed by Isaacs, 1943), citing the lack of demonstrable evidence to suggest that the baby is capable of fantasy formation before the symbolic developments of the toddler phase; rather, naïve cognition and infant temperament are seen as accounting for the infant's subjective experience (Eagle, 2003; Lyon, 2003). Indeed, Stern (1985) postulates the infant as a "perfect recorder of reality," asserting that psychological distortions only occur when compensatory processes are needed to protect security-based needs, such as in the case of the anxiously attached infant. Although psychoanalytic thinkers (e.g., Blum, 2004) acknowledge research that suggests that the baby is pre-adapted to differentiate self from other, many are agnostic about the complete absence of early fantasy, positing the potential for a sense of union with the object, or a feeling of fragmentation during moments of discomfort (e.g., Shuttleworth, 1989; Winnicott, 1960).

Mother–Infant Theories and the Analytic Situation

Theories about the mother–infant relationship have always provided inspiration for re-imagining the analytic situation (e.g., Winnicott, 1960). Abundant research on dyadic interaction has revealed very early patterns of implicit, nonverbal unconscious procedures for how to relate to others (labeled "implicit relational knowing" by Stern et al., 1988); these and related discoveries about the complex conscious and nonconscious states of the mother–infant pair, wherein meaningful experience is mutually constructed, have led to hypothesized links with the co-creative potential of the adult analytic encounter (Tronick, 2003; Harrison & Tronick, 2011). Within this model, which is of particular interest to relational analysts, differentiating and integrating both implicit and explicit modes of intersubjectivity, and grasping the meaning of somatic and linguistic communications are viewed as fundamental, shared activities of the analytic and well as the mother–infant dyad (Lyons-Ruth, 1999; Tronick & Harrison, 2011). A number of theorists caution about extrapolating directly from the infant to the adult mind, stressing the profound differences in levels of cognition (Beebe, Knoblauch, & Rustin, 2003; Tronick, 2003); however, notions of shared mental states, particularly mutual attunement, regulation, and affective reciprocity, derived from knowledge about mother–infant functioning, are proposed as inherent aspects of analytic work.

Initial Stages of Mental Development

Pregnancy and the Maternal Mind

Psychoanalytic theories about pregnancy posit a unique, growth-promoting period in female life wherein profound physical and psychological changes create the potential for emotional development; moreover, the child's progression through distinct psychosexual phases evokes complementary maternal regressions and identifications, facilitating both empathy with the child and openness to personal evolution (Benedek, 1959; Bibring, 1959; Winnicott, 1956, 1971). Contemporary writers stress the pivotal role of the mother's state of mind, beginning in pregnancy, in the quality of the dyad's attachment relationship: re-working the bond with one's own mother and beginning to form emotional connections to the infant are viewed as central tasks for the expectant and new parent (Ammaniti, Tambelli, & Odorisio, 2012; Murray & Cooper, 1997; Stern, 1995). Indeed, the autobiographical narratives and descriptions of mothers in the last trimester of pregnancy suggest distinctive relational patterns and self–other representations that are highly predictive of the emerging mother–infant relationship (Fonagy et al., 1993; Slade & Cohen, 1996).

In Winnicott's (1956) vision of the *primary maternal preoccupation*, the final trimester of pregnancy induces a unique mental state wherein the mother develops a potentially deepened access to the neonate's emotional signals; this special identification with the infant maintains throughout the first weeks of life, the period when the mother's capacity to receive and respond to the infant's states is most needed. Within this model, the newborn's gradual acquisition of mental structure arises in the context of ongoing maternal reverie and caretaking behaviors: The mother's repeated, empathic identifications and interpretations of the infant's shifting states, coupled with her helpful ministrations, transforms the child's bodily discomfort or distress into modulated, less immediate versions of the original experience; these more tolerable forms are internalized, leading to the creation of mental representations of somatic and affective states (Bion, 1962; Winnicott, 1960). From a contemporary, neurobiological perspective the parent's mature brain facilitates the development of the infant's neural systems (Balbernie, 2001).

The mother's unconscious conflicts and fantasies ("ghosts in the nursery"), evoked by the infant's dependency and myriad unique qualities, can intrude into the mother–infant relationship, disrupting her capacity to identify with and reflect on the child's needs (Fraiberg, Adelson, & Shapiro, 1975). Distortions in the interpretation of the infant's cues may result from impairments in the mother's self-regulatory abilities and her failure to differentiate between her own and the baby's mental states (Fonagy et al., 1993; Slade & Cohen, 1996). Such deficits in maternal mirroring contribute to the development of a "false self" wherein the mother's needs effectively dominate and mask the infant's individuality and potential (Winnicott, 1960). Although attachment research has tended to minimize the role of infant endowment in the quality of the dyad's bond, we share the interest of most psychoanalysts in the baby's unique constitutional qualities, and in the complex interplay between these and maternal fantasy; such features as gender, rate of development, and temperament (variations in the child's sleeping and eating patterns, tendencies toward under or over arousal, activity level, sensory vulnerabilities), together with the parental responses that they elicit, form a "basic core" of potential developmental trends (Weil, 1970).

The mother's empathy and self-reflection are correlated with the infant's attachment security as well as with the older child's overall social and emotional functioning, forming an enduring, intergenerational link between the mother's and child's relational and self-regulatory patterns (Fonagy et al., 1993). Contemporary research suggests that the mother's "mind-mindedness"—that is, her capacity to relate to the child as a differentiated individual with a unique mind and separate needs—is a powerful predictor of secure attachment; in the first months of life, mind-mindedness is behaviorally demonstrated in the mother's response to subtle changes in the baby's actions, such as following a shift in the direction of the child's gaze, or imitating the infant's gestures (Meins et al., 2003).

Extensive research on maternal attachment has yielded four distinct relational patterns; mothers' emotional self-reflection and narrative coherence (i.e., capacity to meaningfully integrate affects and interpersonal events) are assessed via the Adult Attachment Interview, which elicits memories about childhood bonds as well as current attitudes toward the baby and other important relationships (Main, 2000; Main & Hesse, 1990; Main, Kaplan, & Cassidy, 1985). The following categories have been delineated: "Secure-Autonomous," marked by the mother's capacity for emotional reflection and availability, along with recognition of the infant's subjectivity; "Dismissive," wherein affective experience of self and baby is denied and there is overall "derogation of thinking and feeling" (Fonagy & Target, 2007, p. 441); "Preoccupied," characterized by the mother's overwhelmed emotional reactions and immersion in past relational conflicts; and "Unresolved," in which the mother, often presenting a history of loss or trauma, manifests poorly organized regulatory strategies. These maternal patterns[1] are highly correlated with infant attachment quality; moreover, "Unresolved," maternal attachment is a known predictor of developmental psychopathology and has been linked to disruptive and dissociative disorders in children and adolescents (Hesse & Main, 2000). Recent work (Ammaniti, Tombelli, & Odorisio, 2012) replicates these findings on maternal attachment, suggesting that the Integrated/Balanced parent, like the Secure-Autonomous mother of previous studies, differentiates between her own and the infant's mind, tolerates emotional arousal and spontaneity, and produces affectively integrated narratives of relational experience; "Restricted" or "Ambivalent" (linked to the Dismissive and Preoccupied categories, respectively) mothers tend toward rigid or confused, contradictory representations of self and child, and manifest narrative styles that are characterized by disruption and incoherence.

Early Mother–Infant Interaction

Contemporary theories posit the neonate's mind as an open, self-organizing system in continuous interaction with the environment (Bornstein et al., 2006; Gergely, 2000; Tronick & Harrison, 2011); perhaps most importantly, the infant is innately motivated to seek maternal contact (Bowlby, 1958) and is uniquely "attuned to other minds" (Stern & The Boston Change Process Study Group, 2004, p. 648). From the outset, the newborn functions as an active meaning-maker, exploring the environment and extracting invariant properties from the social world in order to create generalizations and make predictions (Gergely, 2000; Stern, 1985). Indeed, the infant's innate, active orientation toward language, inherent attunement to parental speech, coordination of vocalizations and facial expressions, and early abilities to discern phonetic distinctions raise the question of whether the first months of life can be accurately described as "pre-verbal" (Litowitz, 2011; Parlade & Iverson, 2011; Vivona, 2012). Historic empirical focus on the baby's apprehension of the physical world, through sensorimotor processes (e.g., Piaget, 1954), has been largely superseded by a prevailing interest in the infant's rather remarkable interpersonal and communicative capacities.

The neonate's inborn attunements and abilities, in combination with the mother's mirroring functions and physical care, give meaning to the earliest bodily and psychological states and result in the gradual mentalization of experience (Bion, 1959, 1962; Fonagy & Target, 2007; Winnicott, 1960). Freud's theorizing about the body-ego, and his notion that early ego structure arises at the border of bodily experience, captures the centrality of close physical contact in the ongoing, dyadic process of communication; his visions of the infant as a closed, autoerotic, and objectless system are clearly outmoded, but conceptualizations of the infant's sense of omnipotence, and of "autistic" and "symbiotic" states may be seen as having some relevance for the baby's initial interest in high levels of *contingent responsiveness* during the first three months of life (Freud, 1914, 1923; Gergely, 2000; Mahler, Pine, & Bergman, 1975). Contemporary views of the infant's mental development conceptualize the mother's relatedness as forms of contingency that facilitate the establishment of primary representations of the bodily and affective self.

Responsive physical care and *marked* affective mirroring (slightly altered, playful transformations of the infant's distress, such as a mock sad face) provide the baby with a sense of causal control and efficacy over physical and psychological states, leading to decreased helplessness and the gradual differentiation of the self and emotional experience (Gergely, 2000).

From the outset, the mother–child pair functions as a mutually regulating "dyadic system" (Beebe, 2005). By around three months of age, most infants manifest greater state regulation and stability; more consistent periods of alertness and increasing overall social responsiveness, including social smiling, create a unique availability for face-to-face interactions that are internalized by the infant (Stern, 1985). There is substantial evidence that implicit, unconscious relational patterns with accompanying affects are established very early in the first year of life (Beebe & Lachmann, 2002; Stern et al., 1988); indeed, young infants detect changes in the mother's usual manner of face-to-face relating, reacting with distress and disconnection when she evinces an unresponsive demeanor (Tronick et al., 1978). Within attachment theory, the baby's increasingly stable, complex, and organized representations of self and other in a relationship are conceived as *internal working models*, cognitive-emotional mental schemas that reflect repeated, internalized mother–child interactions. When the baby is subjected to repeated negative social experience, internal working models tend to rigidify and organize around a sense of hopelessness or inadequacy. These models guide patterns of interpersonal defense and emotional self-regulation, which are observable and measurable by the end of infancy (see the section on *patterns of attachment*). Thoughts and feelings that threaten to disrupt the mother–child relationship are defensively excluded from consciousness; later in development, these defensive processes result in the disjointed and incoherent narratives that insecurely attached children and adults tend to produce when describing interpersonal situations (Main, 1991).

Separation–Individuation and the Older Infant

Separation–individuation encompasses two complementary but distinct processes that reverberate throughout life: the infant's increasing intrapsychic awareness of physical and mental separateness from the mother, as well as the development and expression of unique individual and autonomous qualities (the child's desire for exploration and emerging cognitive, language, and motoric capacities) both begin to unfold at around six months of age (Mahler, Pine, & Bergman, 1975). The baby's dawning realization of self–other differentiation ("hatching") leads to the emergence of the first transitional, "not-me" objects and phenomena (Winnicott, 1953). Moreover, increased differentiation induces the first of two separation crises (the second, during the rapprochement phase of toddlerhood, is discussed in detail in the next chapter): at around seven to nine months of age, manifestations of stranger and separation anxiety reflect a clearer distinction between the mother and other individuals, and greater sensitivity to her comings and goings (Mahler, Pine, & Bergman, 1975).

The infant's sense of separateness is accompanied by new levels of affective sharing within the dyad. The mother functions as a *beacon of emotional orientation* during the final months of infancy, as the baby's enhanced cognitive and motoric capacities facilitate active investigation of the environment (Mahler, 1952). Repeatedly, the newly crawling child ventures out into the world, propelled by the desire to explore, play, and learn, but returns to her side for emotional refueling. During brief periods of physical separation from the mother's body, such distal modes of communication as visual sharing and showing toys, vocalizations, and the first one-word utterances serve as means for maintaining connection.

At around seven to nine months, "infants gradually come upon the momentous realization that inner subjective experiences, the 'subject matter' of the mind, are potentially shareable..." (Stern, 1985, p. 124). The emergence of *joint attention*—that is, the capacity to coordinate attention between the self, the mother and an external object or event—represents a new dimension of dyadic reciprocity and represents a critical step toward eventual social capacities, such as the ability to talk about mental states (Kristen et al., 2011). Moreover, the older infant actively seeks out the mother's mental state, then uses her emotional cues to guide personal reactions; this process, known as *social referencing*, has been empirically illustrated via the "visual cliff" experiment: An infant crawling across a surface hesitates when a perceived dropoff is encountered, looks to the mother, and crosses the "cliff" only if she evinces an encouraging, reassuring demeanor (Sorce et al., 1985). Social referencing functions as an early forerunner of superego development; although it predates the parent's deliberate efforts at socialization and the child's sense of personal wrongdoing, it is a preliminary form of parent–infant emotional communication that directly impacts the infant's behavior.

Patterns of Attachment

Although separation–individuation theory envisions the mother as a beacon of emotional orientation, attachment theory employs the concept of the "secure base" to describe the older infant's physical and affective reliance on maternal proximity. Activation of the attachment system—as a result of conditions that engender the baby's anxiety and felt insecurity—leads to renewed seeking of maternal contact for comfort and soothing, a process that is considered foundational for the development of emotional self-regulation. Indeed, secure attachment experiences are crucial for the establishment of brain-based self-regulatory mechanisms that allow the older child to tolerate interpersonal stress, sustain attention, and develop capacities to interpret others' mental states (Balbernie, 2001; Fonagy, 2002; Shore, 1999).

Measurable aspects of secure base behavior, such as the baby's forays into independent exploration, manifest distress and contact-seeking, are captured in the "Strange Situation," a renowned research tool that uses a series of brief maternal separations and reunions to engender the baby's anxiety and provoke attachment behaviors (Ainsworth et al., 1978). Results of the original Strange Situation study delineate three categories of infant attachment: "Secure," in which children play freely in their mother's presence, manifest distress at her absence, and find comfort in her return; "Avoidant," which describes children who evince neutral and ostensibly unruffled attitudes during separation and reunion; and "Ambivalent/Resistant" children, who are marked by a high level of distress at all points during the experiment, including a failure to be comforted by the mother's return. These three classifications correspond, respectively, with the maternal designations of Autonomous, Dismissive, and Preoccupied. A fourth category, "Disorganized/Disoriented," characterized by the child's contradictory and incompatible behaviors upon reunion with the mother, such as approaching and then freezing, or smiling while hitting, was later developed; like the corresponding maternal category of "Unresolved," this pattern of attachment has been linked to developmental pathology (Hesse & Main, 2000).[2]

A number of theorists have attempted to integrate patterns of attachment with psychoanalytic models. Sandler (2003) relates the attachment categories to his own notion of the "role relationship," wherein each member of a dyad unconsciously affects the other in an effort to evoke a desired response. In his view, the individual seeks to recreate security feelings associated with the original parental objects, via unconscious fantasy and acting on the external world, throughout the life span. Toward this end, children modify and control their perceptions, employing whatever age-appropriate ego capacities are available, in order to achieve a sense of security and mitigate anxiety. (He cites the "avoidant" child's heavy reliance on denial of affect as an example.) Diamond (2004) connects the un-integrated, contradictory internal schemes and behaviors of the "disorganized" infant with Melanie Klein's emphasis on the use of splitting and projection to manage persecutory anxieties. Links between the concept of object constancy (a stable, internalized connection to the parent) and the securely attached child suggest that mental representation of the mother as a secure base fosters the capacity to evoke her image as a soothing and self-regulating presence (e.g., Eagle, 2003). Winnicott's (1960) notion of the "false self vividly portrays the dilemma of the insecurely attached infant, whose attempts to comply with maternal defensiveness and projections requires that he or she "distort and obliterate" (Slade, 2000, p. 1157) personal needs in order to maintain the parent–child bond.

The Transition to the Toddler Phase

The older infant's preoccupation with motor skills, during the aptly named "practicing phase" (Mahler, 1972), and the seemingly relentless pursuit of upright mobility leads to a temporary diminishment of concern with maternal proximity. Many infants evince a single-minded focus on walking and appear impervious to minor bumps and falls. The exhilaration of the newly walking infant/toddler is represented by Mahler's (1972) assertion that "the world is his oyster." Nonetheless, a sudden awareness of maternal absence leads to low-keyed reactions. As children enter the toddler phase, increased realization of self–other differentiation and distance induces a second wave of separation anxiety, wherein the mother's presence is sought with renewed vigor. Olesker's (1990) observation of gender differences led her to hypothesize that girls' more precocious awareness of self–other differentiation and greater sensitivity to maternal mental states may predispose them to anxiety and more muted exuberance during the practicing period. In her view, mothers evince less ambivalent support for their male infants' autonomy and physical accomplishments.

The child's cognitive and linguistic maturation leads to a vast expansion of dyadic communication, including the emergence of symbolic functions such as early forms of language, imitation, and play. Significantly increased verbal comprehension and the beginning expression of one-word phrases transforms the mother–infant relationship; as experience is increasingly subject to verbal mediation, the previous intimacy of the dyad's bodily contact is gradually replaced by more distal methods of affective sharing.

Summary

Contemporary psychoanalytic, attachment, and neurobiological theories posit infancy as a crucial period for the establishment of relational and self-regulatory mental structures. Attachment theory has guided a generation of infant studies and led to revitalization and revision of psychoanalytic thinking; moreover, fascination with baby-watching and with the mother–child dyad has led a number of theorists to posit connections between the mother–infant dyad and the shared subjectivities of the analytic situation.

Early mental development is facilitated by maternal reverie and mirroring functions, which serve to receive, interpret, and transform the baby's immediate physical and psychological experience, leading to representations of the bodily and affective self. The mother–infant relationship functions as a dyadic system in which mutual affective sharing and regulation are dominant forms of communication. As the infant gains awareness of mother and self differentiation, and cognitive, linguistic, and motoric abilities emerge, new modes of relating (e.g., joint attention and social referencing) are possible; during the latter portion of infancy, the mother functions as a beacon of emotional orientation during the child's initial forays into exploration and mastery of the environment. By the end of the first year, the infant displays stable patterns of attachment and self-regulatory tendencies. As infancy draws to a close, the baby becomes preoccupied with the developmental task of walking. The achievement of upright mobility marks the shift into toddlerhood.

The following points are particularly relevant for working with infants and mothers:

- In the first months of life, maternal reverie and contingent responsiveness are essential elements of dyadic bonding which facilitate the baby's gradual development of internal, emotional self-regulatory functions. The mother's psychological states and her quality of relationships are key determinants of infant developmental outcome.

- The infant's unique qualities, along with maternal responsiveness and early mother–infant interaction, form the basis for the baby's mental representations of relationships; these are increasingly organized and consolidated over the course of infancy, and yield stable behavioral patterns of attachment by the end of the first year of life.
- The emergence of joint attention and social referencing, in the last quarter of the infant year, signal a heightened sense of self–other differentiation and a new capacity for affective, intersubjective sharing. The mother serves as a "beacon of emotional orientation" and a "secure base": The baby is motivated to explore the environment but seeks frequent contact, often returning to her side for emotional refueling.
- As the baby transitions to the toddler phase of development, the drive to achieve upright mobility temporarily dominates the child's experience.

Notes

1. A meta-review by Bakermans-Kranenburg and Van Ijzendoor (2009) reveals the following distribution for nonclinical, American mothers: Autonomous, 58%; Dismissive, 23%; Preoccupied, 19%; 18% were further classified as Unresolved. Moreover, Van ijzendoorn (1995) found 75% continuity from maternal to baby for designation of secure or insecure attachment.

2. In nonclinical samples, the proportions of these categories are reported to be the following: 62% Secure, 15% Avoidant, 9% Resistant, and 15 % Disorganized (Van Ijzendoorn, Scheungel, & Bakermans-Kranenburg, 1999).

References

Ackerman, S. (2010). Is infant research useful in clinical work with adults? *Journal of the American Psychoanalytic Association, 58,* 1201–1211.

Ainsworth, M. D. S., Blehar, M. C., Waters, E., & Wall, S. (1978). *Patterns of Attachment: a Psychological Study of the Strange Situation.* Hillsdale, NJ: Erlbaum.

Ammaniti, M., Tambelli, R., & Odorisio, F (2013). Exploring maternal representations during pregnancy in normal and at-risk samples: the use of the interview of maternal representations during pregnancy. *Infant Mental Health Journal, 34,* 1–10.

Bakermans-Kranenburg, M. J., & Van Ijzendoor, M. H. (2009). The first 10,000 adult attachment interviews: distribution of adult attachment representations in clinical and non-clinical groups. *Attachment and Human Development, 11,* 223–263.

Balbernie, R. (2001). Circuits and circumstances: the neurobiological consequences of early relationship experiences and how they shape later behavior. *Journal of Child Psychotherapy, 27,* 237–255.

Beebe, B. (2005). Mother-infant research informs mother-infant treatment. *Psychoanalytic Study of the Child, 60,* 7–46.

Beebe, B., Knoblauch, S., & Rustin, J. (2003). Introduction: a systems view. *Psychoanalytic Dialogues, 13,* 743–775.

Beebe, B. & Lachmann, F. (2002). Organizing principles of interaction from infant research and the lifespan prediction of attachment: application to adult treatment. *Journal of Infant, Child and Adolescent Psychotherapy, 2,* 61–89.

Benedek, T. (1959). Parenthood as a developmental phase—a contribution to the libido theory. *Journal of the American Psychoanalytic Association, 7,* 389–417.

Bibring, G. (1959). Some considerations of the psychological processes in pregnancy. *Psychoanalytic Study of the Child, 14,* 113–121.

Bick, E. (1964). Notes on infant observation in psychoanalytic training. *International Journal of Psychoanalysis, 45,* 558–566.

Bion, W. R. (1959). Attacks on linking. *International Journal of Psychoanalysis, 40,* 308–315.

Bion, W. R. (1962). *Learning from Experience.* London: Heinemann.

Blum, H. P. (2004). Separation-individuation theory and attachment theory. *Journal of the American Psychoanalytic Association, 52,* 535–553.

Bornstein, M. H., Hahn, C., Bell, C., Haynes, O. M., Slater, A., Golding, J., et al. (2006). Stability in cognition across early childhood: a developmental cascade. *Psychological Science, 17,* 151–158.

Bowlby, J. (1958). The nature of the child's tie to his mother. *International Journal of Psycho-Analysis, 39,* 350–373.

Bowlby, J. (1969). *Attachment and Loss, Vol. 1: Attachment.* London: Hogarth Press and the Institute of Psycho-Analysis.

Bowlby, J. (1973). *Attachment and Loss, Vol. 2: Separation: Anxiety and Anger.* London: Hogarth Press and the Institute of Psycho-Analysis.

Diamond, D. (2004). Attachment disorganization: the reunion of attachment theory and psychoanalysis. *Psychoanalytic Psychology, 21,* 276–299.

Eagle, M. (2003). Clinical implications of attachment theory. *Psychoanalytic Inquiry, 23,* 27–53.

Fonagy, P (2001). *Psychoanalysis and Attachment Theory.* New York: Other Press.

Fonagy, P. (2002). The internal working model or the interpersonal interpretive function. *Journal of Infant, Child and Adolescent Psychotherapy, 2,* 27–38.

Fonagy, P., Steele, M., Moran, G., Steele, H., & Higgitt, A. (1993). Measuring the ghost in the nursery: an empirical study of the relation between parents' mental representations of childhood experience and their infants' security of attachment. *Journal of the American Psychoanalytic Association, 41,* 957–989.

Fonagy, P. & Target, M. (2002). Early intervention and the development of self-regulation. *Psychoanalytic Inquiry 22,* 307–335.

Fonagy, P. & Target, M. (2007). Playing with reality: IV: A theory of external reality rooted in intersubjectivity. *International Journal of Psychoanalysis, 88,* 917-938.

Fraiberg, S., Adelson, E., & Shapiro, V. (1975). Ghosts in the nursery: a psychoanalytic approach to the problem of impaired infant-mother relationships. *Journal of the American Academy of Child Psychiatry, 14,* 387–421.

Freud, A. (1953). Some remarks on infant observation. In *The Writings of Anna Freud* (Vol. *IV*). New York: International Universities Press.

Freud, S. (1914). On narcissism: an introduction. In James Strachey (Ed. & Trans.) *The Standard Edition of the Complete Works of Sigmund Freud* (Vol. *14*). London: Hogarth Press.

Freud, S. (1923). The ego and the id. In James Strachey (Ed. and Trans.) *The Standard Edition of the Complete Works of Sigmund Freud* (Vol. *19*). London: Hogarth Press.

Gergely, G. (2000). Reapproaching Mahler: new perspectives on normal autism, symbiosis, splitting and libidinal object constancy from cognitive developmental theory. *Journal of the American Psychoanalytic Association, 48,* 1197–1228.

Green, A. (2000). What kind of research for psychoanalysis? In J. Sander, A. Sandler, & R. Davies (Eds.), *Clinical and Observational Psychoanalytic Research: Roots of a Controversy.* Madison, CT: International Universities Press.

Harpaz-Rotem, I. & Bergman, A. (2006). On an evolving theory of attachment: rapprochement—theory of a developing mind. *Psychoanalytic Study of the Child, 61,* 170–189.

Harrison, A. & Tronick, E. (2011). "The noise monitor": a developmental perspective on verbal and nonverbal meaning-making in psychoanalysis. *Journal of the American Psychoanalytic Association, 59, 961-982.*

Hesse, E. & Main, M. (2000). Disorganized infant, child and adult attachment: collapse in behavioral and attentional strategies. *Journal of the American Psychoanalytic Association, 48,* 1097–1127.

Hug-Hellmuth, H. Von (1919). *A Study of the Mental Life of the Child.* Washington, DC: Nervous and Mental Diseases Publishing Company.

Isaacs, S. (1943). The nature and function of phantasy. *International Journal of Psychoanalysis, 29,* 73–97.

Kristen, S., Sodian, B., Thoermer, C., & Perst, H. (2011). Infants' joint attention skills predict toddlers' emerging mental state language. *Development Psychology, 47,* 1207–1219.

Litowitz, B. E. (2011). From dyad to dialogue: language and the early relationship in American Psychoanalytic Theory. *Journal of the American Psychoanalytic Association, 59,* 483–507.

Lyon, K. A. (2003). Unconscious fantasy: its scientific status and clinical entity. *Journal of the American Psychoanalytic Association. 51,* 957–967.

Lyons-Ruth, K. (1999). The two-person unconscious: intersubjective dialogues, enactive relational representation and the emergence of new forms of relational organization. *Psychoanalytic Inquiry, 19,* 576–617.

Mahler, M. (1952). On childhood psychosis and schizophrenia—autistic and symbiotic infantile processes. *Psychoanalytic Study of the Child, 7,* 286–305.

Mahler, M. (1963). Thoughts about development and individuation. *Psychoanalytic Study of the Child, 18,* 307–324.

Mahler, M. (1972). On the first three subphases of the separation-individuation process. *International Journal of Psychoanalysis, 53*, 333–338.

Mahler, M., Pine, F., & Bergman, A. (1975). *The Psychological Birth of the Human Infant: Symbiosis and Individuation.* New York: Basic Books.

Main, M. (1991). Metacognitive knowledge, metacognitive monitoring, and singular (coherent) vs. multiple (incoherent) models of attachment. Findings and directions for future research. In C. Parkes, J. Stevenson-Hinde, & P. Marris (Eds.), *Attachment Across the Life Cycle* (pp. 127–160). London: Routledge Press.

Main, M. (2000). The organized categories of infant, child and adult attachment: flexible vs. inflexible attention under attachment-related stress. *Journal of the American Psychoanalytic Association, 48*, 1055–1095.

Main, M. & Hesse, E. (1990). Lack of mourning in adulthood and its relationship to infant disorganization: some speculations regarding causal mechanisms. In M. Greenberg, D. Cicchetti, & M. Cummings (Eds.), *Attachment in the Preschool Years: Theory, Research and Intervention* (pp. 161–182). Chicago: University of Chicago Press.

Main, M., Kaplan, N., & Cassidy, J. (1985). Security in infancy, childhood and adulthood: a move to the level of representation. In E. Bretherton & E. Waters (Eds.), *Growing Points of Attachment Theory and Research.* Monographs of the Society for Research in Child Development, *50*, 66–104.

Meins, E., Fernyhough, C., Wainwright, R., Clark-Carter, D., Gupta, M. D., Fradley, E., et al. (2003). Pathways to understanding mind: construct validity and predictive validity of maternal mind-mindedness. *Child Development, 74*, 1194–1211.

Midgley, N. (2007). Anna Freud: the Hampstead War Nurseries and the role of direct observation of children for psychoanalysis. *International Journal of Psychoanalysis, 88*, 939–959.

Murray, L. & Cooper, P. J. (1997). *Postpartum Depression and Child Development.* New York: Guilford Press.

Olesker, W. (1990). Sex differences during early separation-individuation. *Journal of the American Psychoanalytic Association, 38*, 325–346.

Parlade, M. V. & Iverson, J. M. (2011). The interplay between language, gesture and affect during communicative transition: a dynamic systems approach. *Developmental Psychology, 47*, 820–833.

Piaget, J. (1954). *The Construction of Reality in the Child*. New York: Basic Books.

Sandler, J. (2003). On attachment to internal objects. *Psychoanalytic Inquiry, 23*, 12–26.

Shore, A. (1999). Commentary by Allan N. Shore. *Neuropsychoanalysis, 1*, 49–55.

Shuttleworth, J. (1989). Psychoanalytic theory and infant development. In L. Miller, M. E. Ruskin, M. J. Ruskin, & J. Shuttleworth (Eds.), *Closely Observed Infants* (pp. 22–51). London: Duckworth & Co.

Sorce, J. F., Emde, R. N., Campos, J., & Klinnert, M. (1985). Maternal emotional signaling: its effect on the visual cliff behavior of 1-year-olds. *Developmental Psychology, 21*, 195–200.

Slade, A. (2000). The development and organization of attachment: implications for psychoanalysis. *Journal of the American Psychoanalytic Association, 48*, 1147–1174.

Slade, A. & Cohen, L. (1996). Parenting and the remembrance of things past. *Infant Mental Health Journal, 17*, 217–239.

Spitz, R. (1946). Hospitalism: a follow-up report on an investigation described in Vol. I. *Psychoanalytic Study of the Child, 2*, 113–117.

Stern, D. N. (1985). *The Interpersonal World of the Infant: A View from Psychoanalysis and Developmental Psychology*. New York: Basic Books.

Stern, D. N. (1995). *The Motherhood Constellation: A Unified View of Parent-Infant Psychotherapy*. New York: Basic Books.

Stern, D. N. (2000). The relevance of empirical infant research to psychoanalytic theory and practice. In J. Sandler, A. Sandler, & R. Davies (Eds.), *Clinical and Observational Psychoanalytic Research: Roots of a Controversy* (pp. 73–91). Madison, CT: International Universities Press.

Stern, D. N., Sander, L. W., Nahum, J. P., Harrison, A. M., Lyons-Ruth, K., Morgan, A. C., et al. (1988). Non-interpretive mechanisms in psychoanalytic therapy: the "something more" than interpretation. *International Journal of Psychoanalysis, 79*, 903–921.

Stern, D. N., & The Boston Change Process Study Group. (2004). Some implications of infant observation for psychoanalysis. In A. M. Cooper (Ed.), *Contemporary Psychoanalysis in America: Leading Analysts Present Their Work* (pp. 641–689). Washington, DC: American Psychiatric Publishing.

Tronick, E. Z. (2003). "Of course all relationships are unique": how co-creative processes generate unique mother-infant and patient-therapist relationships and change other relationships. *Psychoanalytic Inquiry, 23,* 473–491.

Tronick, E. Z., Als, H., Adamson, L., Wise, S., & Brazelton, T. B. (1978). The infant's response to entrapment between contradictory messages in face-to-face interaction. *Journal of the American Academy of Child Psychiatry, 17,* 1–13.

Van Ijzendoorn, M. H. (1995). Adult attachment representations, parental responsiveness, and infant attachment: a meta-analysis on the predictive validity of the Adult Attachment Interview. *Psychological Bulletin, 117,* 387–403.

Vivona, J. M. (2012). Is there a nonverbal period of development? *Journal of the American Psychoanalytic Association, 60,* 231–265.

Weil, A. (1970). The basic core. *Psychoanalytic Study of the Child, 25,* 442–460.

Winnicott, D. W. (1953). Transitional objects and transitional phenomena—a study of the first not-me possession. *International Journal of Psychoanalysis, 34,* 89–97.

Winnicott, D. W. (1956). Primary maternal preoccupation. In *Collected Papers, Through Paediatrics to Psycho-analysis* (pp. 300–305). London: Tavistock Publications.

Winnicott, D. W. (1960). The theory of the parent-infant relationship. *International Journal of Psychoanalysis, 41,* 585–595.

Winnicott, D. W. (1975). Through pediatrics to psychoanalysis. *The International Psychoanalytic Library, 100,* 1–325. London: The Hogarth Press.

3

Toddlerhood: Separation– Individuation, Rapprochement, and the Forerunners of Superego Development

Overview

Toddlerhood begins with the achievement of upright mobility, typically at around one year of age, and extends through the third birthday. Once subsumed within the overarching period of pregenital sexual organization, it is now viewed as a distinct phase of early development marked by the child's emerging capacities for self-awareness and the first encounters with socialization. The toddler's psychological achievements include bodily and mental self–other differentiation, language-based communication and imitative play, and internalization of parental standards (Bloom, 1993; Courage & Howe, 2002; Mahler, Pine, & Bergman, 1975; Piaget, 1962a); these attainments are universally recognized as fundamental to an expansion of the child's inner world and to the deepening of personal identity and relationships. Indeed, both empirical and psychoanalytic theorists view the toddler years as defined by critical advances in moral and self-regulatory mental organizations, the forerunners of later superego formation (e.g., Kochanska et al., 2010). The autonomous strivings of the mobile young child, frequently expressed via self-assertive or negative pronouncements and actions in response to growing environmental demands, are among the highly visible behavioral indicators of this phase.

Historical Perspectives

Classic psychoanalytic literature contains few references to toddlerhood as a discrete period of development outside of its concurrence with the anal phase. Traditional theory assumes an inevitable upsurge of anal erogeneity that dominates the toddler's object relations, subjecting them to dramatic alternations between libidinous and aggressive–sadistic urges; bodily products, most notably feces, are experienced as valuable possessions, and their retention and expulsion are only reluctantly submitted to parental control (A. Freud, 1936). Central tasks of this period, such as transformation of anal erotic instincts into psychic structure and the child's achievement of "sphincter-morality" (Ferenczi, 1925), are conceptualized as necessary precursors to *ego ideal* (see glossary) and superego development (Freud, 1917; Shengold, 1985). The child's first encounters with active socialization, via maternal demands for bowel and bladder management, contribute to the emergence of essential defenses—repression, reaction formation, identification with the aggressor—which help neutralize sadistic and erotic urges, and give rise to such trends as cleanliness, orderliness, and fastidiousness (Sandler & Freud, 1983).

Although clearly anchored in a single psychosexual etiology, and heavily derived from hypotheses about adult psychopathology, these original formulations nonetheless capture the universally acknowledged mother–toddler shared preoccupation with the child's bodily functions and products. Moreover, conceptualizations of the child's central dilemma, that is, resolving adult demands with personal pleasure seeking, and of the resultant process of self-regulatory structuralization are highly consistent with contemporary views of this phase as instrumental for the development of morality and self-control.

Mahler's (1972) theory of *rapprochement* (described in the next section), with its emphasis on the child's emerging sense of separateness and concomitant anxieties, expanded the traditional psychoanalytic view of the toddler beyond specific anal phase conflicts. She contextualized the child's struggles within the maternal relationship; moreover, a broader scope of cognitive, motoric, and linguistic capacities was granted a pivotal role in toddler development. Within the separation–individuation model, the toddler's basic tasks include the gradual renunciation of symbiotic omnipotence and acceptance of reality. Acquisition of a unified intrapsychic representation of the object relationship (*libidinal object constancy*) is a defining developmental achievement for the pre-oedipal child that scaffolds the emergence of higher-level self-regulatory structures. Contemporary empirical work supports Mahler's notions of the mother's needed availability, self-restraint, and consistency in the face of the toddler's inevitable negativistic and ambivalent attitudes. For example, studies in the development of conscience demonstrate that maternal provision of supportive rather than punitive reactions is correlated with the attainment of age-appropriate behavioral self-control (Laible & Thompson, 2002; Spinrad et al., 2007).

Mahler's vision of the crucial role of rapprochement in mental development, her belief in the lifelong human struggle between autonomy and intimacy, and her view of object constancy as an open-ended achievement inspired certain theorists to link the toddler's inner struggles with later developmental conflicts. For example, Blos's (1967) adolescent theory, described in some detail in chapter 6, draws upon the model of early separation–individuation to address the pubescent child's autonomous strivings and fears of re-engulfment in the infantile parent–child relationship. Moreover, Mahler (1972) and others (e.g., Masterson & Rinsley, 1975) posited potential continuity between the rapprochement crisis, characterized by the child's abandonment anxiety and poor affect tolerance, and the later emergence of borderline psychopathology. Contemporary views of development largely reject linearity between early and later phases, but the central developmental tasks of rapprochement—establishment of capacities for inner rather than external conflict, stable internal representations, and expansion of resources for emotional self-control—are considered foundational for the child's progressive development.

Rapprochement and Separation–Individuation

In the period between 15 and 22 months, the child's increased awareness of self–other differentiation leads to a resurgence of separation anxiety and a renewed demand for maternal proximity (Mahler, 1972; Mahler, Pine, & Bergman, 1975). There is a notable decline in the apparent sense of imperviousness and grandiosity that the newly walking toddler displays; in its place, a low-keyed quality dominates the child's mood. Urgent shadowing of the mother, with manifest attempts to control her whereabouts, reflect a triad of anxieties—loss of the parent, withdrawal of parental approval, and castration—which are amplified by the parent's demands for behavioral self-control, the toddler's increased sensitivity to adults' reactions and standards, and a heightened awareness of the body, particularly of anal and urethral pressures. At the apex of the rapprochement phase, the child's mounting fears of object loss and injury vie with more progressive drives toward autonomy; the "rapprochement crisis" ensues, wherein distressed inner states and contradictory urges suffuse the toddler's behavior. Ultimately, the struggles of this phase are resolved with the acquisition of a capacity for libidinal object constancy, marked by enduring, internalized representations of self and other that retain their positive qualities despite negative affective states and situational vagaries (Gergely, 2000; McDevitt, 1975).

Underlying Developments in Self-Awareness and Identity

Mahler's systematic observations of mother–child dyads predated the vast contemporary reservoir of empirical research; nonetheless, her assumptions about the toddler's intensified awareness of a separate self, and the concomitant sensitivities to maternal disapproval and potential bodily injury, presage major experimental findings about toddler development. In the latter half of the second year, the child acquires knowledge of the self as a separate, unique, and recognizable entity; the attainment of a categorical self-concept is empirically demonstrated via mirror self-recognition and referral to the self via language and pointing (Lewis & Brooks-Gunn, 1979). The subsequent emergence of self-aware emotions, such as shame and pride, and increased capacities to compare and measure the self against external standards are reflected by the toddler's expression of distress when caught in violation of a behavioral norm, or in negative reactions to broken or missing items (Emde, Johnson, & Easterbrooks, 1987; Stipek, Gralinski, & Koop, 1990). More complex aspects of self-knowledge and identity, such as gender, are informed by the toddler's naïve cognition, including highly concrete self–other comparisons. Individual subjectivity is only partially grasped, but the toddler is increasingly aware of personal feelings, goals, and preferences; the mother's expanding efforts at socialization and her selective disapproval reinforces differentiation between the parent's and child's mental states, between her ambitions and the toddler's wishes (Harpez-Rotem & Bergman, 2006).

Basic knowledge about sex differences and gender-based identity emerges by the age of two years. Toddlers label themselves as male or female and manifest keen interest in anatomical differences. However, they employ concrete clues, such as hair length and manner of dress, to determine gender categories (Martin & Ruble, 2004; Senet, 2004). Classical psychoanalytic theories emphasize the link between the young child's discovery of sex differences and the inevitable emergence of castration anxiety; in the case of the girl, feelings of bodily and personal inadequacy ensue (e.g., Olesker, 1998). However, contemporary research has necessitated a reconceptualization of certain bedrock assumptions, such as the ubiquity of the girl's penis envy. It is now acknowledged that before the age of three, children do not automatically connect gender with genitals. Moreover, both boys and girls tend to manifest positive affects in regard to their own sex (DeMarneffe, 1997; Senet, 2004). We support an integration of these positions: As many clinical and more casual observers of toddlers can attest, avid curiosity about the genitals, transient but intense fears about bodily and genital injury, and envious reactions to the body that the opposite sex possesses are extremely common. Moreover, the physical realities of female anatomy (specifically the proximity of the genital to the anus) predispose the girl, especially during the period of toilet training, toward the sense of her genital as dirty (Gilmore, 1998). The toddler's sensitivity to objects that are broken or incomplete is not limited to the inanimate world and informs reactions to bodily differences. When considered in the context of children's egocentric and concrete thinking, it is not surprising that they suffer from castration fears, or feelings and fantasies that something is missing or has been lost. Of course, such experiences are more likely to accrue meaning and become linked with enduring self-fantasies when they are reinforced by toddlers' perceptions of parental attitudes or their literal interpretations of serendipitous events, or when subsequent phases of development pose challenges to the sense of bodily integrity and self-worth.

Conflict and Ambivalence during Rapprochement

As the milestone of walking is practiced and achieved, the toddler evinces a sense of elation that is perhaps best captured by Mahler's (1972) observation that "the world is his oyster" or Greenacre's (1957) reference to a "love affair with the world." A palpable deflation evolves by around 15 months, arising from a confluence of developments that include the following: the child's experience of greater physical separation, fueled by mobility; an awareness of separate mental states, augmented by increasing exposure to maternal demands that clash with the toddler's personal desires; the imposition of societal expectations, transmitted via the parent, for self-discipline and physical self-control; the advent of more distal, language-based communications with the mother and the concomitant decline of the dyad's bodily intimacy; and the encroachment of other reality-based obstacles upon the toddler's sense of magical omnipotence (Bergman & Harpez-Rotem, 2004; Mahler, 1972; Milrod, 1982; Stern, 1985). Renewed separation anxiety and desire for the mother's presence are conflictual, however, as they vie with the child's pleasure in autonomy and independent action. The result is the expression of "ambitendency," mother-directed behaviors that are marked by their alternately clinging and rejecting nature (Mahler & McDevitt, 1968; Mahler, Pine, & Bergman, 1975; Meissner, 2009).

Although most psychoanalytic thinkers consider the toddler's mixed signals as normative, and largely as internally generated, attachment theorists caution against assuming the inevitability of ambivalent attitudes. These writers (e.g., Lyons-Ruth, 1991) emphasize ongoing attachment and mutual emotional regulation, rather than separation, as dominant tasks for the toddler period. They point to the confusing, approach-avoidant behaviors that are routinely observed in anxiously attached mother–toddler pairs as a reflection of the dyad's poorly organized systems of affective reciprocity and communication. While acknowledging the link of such behavioral manifestations with insecure attachment, we take a fairly routine psychoanalytic view toward the developmental emergence of conflict and ambivalence in toddlerhood, assuming that even well-functioning dyads nonetheless are buffeted by the child's emerging selfhood and concomitant internal disequilibrium, the mother's unique response to the loss of the infancy experience infancy, and the pressures placed on both by her shifting role toward transmitter of societal regulations.

Although not all theorists subscribe to the view of ubiquitous inner conflict and ambivalence, the toddler's commonly observed, outward displays of oppositionality and negativism are almost universally acknowledged. Resistant behaviors, and the child's famously liberal usage of the word "no," reflect autonomous strivings and reinforce self–other differentiation (Mahler, Pine, & Bergman, 1975; Spitz, 1957). Empirical findings suggest very high normative rates of mother–toddler conflict, typically occurring multiple times per hour (Laible & Thompson, 2002). Moreover, the toddler's protests and failures of compliance are generally viewed as manifestations of developmental trends, such as self-assertion and independence, rather than problematic parenting or poor dyadic relations (Dix et al., 2007; Laible, Panfile, & Makariev, 2008).

Superego Development during the Toddler Phase

Contemporary psychoanalytic and empirical views of super-ego development suggest that forerunners emerge during the first months of life, as manifestations of affective reciprocity and mutual regulation in the mother–infant relationship. Hallmarks of inter-subjectivity, such as social referencing in the latter part of the first year, demonstrate the baby's internalization of parental reactions and prohibitions as well as an early capacity to incorporate those as a guide for personal behavior. During the toddler period, with its proliferation of symbolic capacities and unprecedented level of self-awareness, these largely nonverbal processes undergo considerable transformation. Language, imitation, and play create multiple venues for more complex identifications with adult standards and behaviors. Moreover, the child's level of self–other differentiation and verbal comprehension facilitate a greater awareness of others' needs and expectations and a wider range of potential responsiveness. Self-conscious emotions, self-evaluative capacities, and heightened sensitivity to parental approbation motivate the toddler toward self-regulation and conciliatory actions that tend to elicit parental praise and ultimately contribute to positive self-regard. As the rapprochement phase proceeds, the toddler's primary anxiety about object loss shifts from concern about the mother's proximity to anticipated loss of her approval. The inevitable tensions and inner discomforts that the toddler endures, as his or her impulses are increasingly subject to parental judgment, are essential steps in the gradual internalization of moral conflicts and the child's progression toward an inner set of self-generated controls, punishments, and rewards (Kennedy & Yorke, 1982).

Within the empirical literature, toddlerhood is widely conceived as the phase in which the conscience system, which is theorized to comprise both moral emotions (e.g., guilt, empathy) and ethical conduct, begins to emerge. The presence of moral behavioral indicators in the second year of life, such as empathic gestures and attempts at self-restraint in the absence of the parent, robustly predicts behavioral self-control and prosocial gestures in later childhood (Kochanska et al., 2010). Developmental theorists posit the gradual establishment of an inner moral identity, originating in the toddler phase, which functions as the child's internal guide and directs future actions. A sense of a moral self is empirically demonstrated, by around the age of three years, via the child's expressed concrete notions of right versus wrong, helpful responding to another's distress and manifest affective discomfort during wrongdoing (Buchsbaum & Emde, 1990; Emde et al., 1991; Vaish, Missana, & Tomasello, 2011).

Post-Freudian psychoanalytic conceptions of moral development similarly identify the emergence of superego precursors during the toddler months, significantly before oedipal phase resolutions (Holder, 1982); these include such phenomena as identification with the aggressor (Sandler & Freud, 1983), the *wished-for self-image* (Milrod, 1982), and Sandler's (1960) notion of "pre-autonomous superego schemes," which he posits as "...a sort of undergraduate superego which only works under the supervision of the parents" (p. 152). The toddler's enhanced sense of separateness and the accompanying felt loss of the parent–child union create an intense desire to achieve a likeness to the parent, accomplished via imitation and other forms of identification with adult standards and actions. Such strivings can be hypothesized as an early form of the ego ideal (e.g., Jacobson, 1954; Milrod, 1982). In distinction to empirical writers, however, most psychoanalysts see meaningful differences between the concrete, typically self-aggrandizing and shame-driven quality of the toddler's superego precursors and the older, postoedipal child's more autonomous manifestations of guilt and moral anxiety.

We find substantial heuristic value in Milrod's (1982) unique conceptualization of the wished-for self-image, which captures the toddler's intense drive toward concrete, action-based identifications with admired parental qualities; these are largely enacted through deferred imitation, a cognitive hallmark of the toddler phase (Piaget, 1952). Elaborating on Jacobson's (1954) distinctions between the ego ideal and the wishful self-concept, Milrod (1982,

2002) postulates the emergence of the latter during the rapprochement period, as the exhilaration of the practicing phase comes to an end and toddler gains greater awareness of self–other differentiation. The narcissistic injury of lost self–mother merger and grandiosity triggers a longing for similarity to the parent. No longer gratified by a sense of magical control over the mother, the child begins to strive for concrete likenesses. Identification with the parent's activities and attributes provides compensation for the toddler's sense of loss and powerlessness. The wished-for self-image is conceptualized as a precursor to superego development, and is distinguished from later internalizations of the parents' more abstract standards and values during the oedipal phase.

As Milrod's theory suggests, the toddler relies on positive parental identifications as well as prohibitions for the establishment of self-regulatory structures; together, these serve as forerunners of the self-rewarding and self-punitive functions of the more mature superego. Esteem-enhancing aspects of the developing superego represent loved and admired qualities of the parent. Overly hostile and rigid parental superego functioning may lead to retaliatory and harsh reactions, disrupting the child's early efforts toward self-regulation and limiting opportunities for positive internalizations (Schafer, 1960). Contemporary research upholds this view, emphasizing ongoing maternal warmth and acceptance, as well as support for the toddler's autonomy, as crucial factors in the emergence of moral conscience. Secure attachment to the parent is seen as freeing up mental focus, which allows the child to concentrate on developmental tasks (e.g., storing transmitted values and standards in semantic memory) rather than on attachment-based anxieties (Kochanska et al., 2004; Kochanska et al., 2010). Half a century earlier, Mahler's (1963) parent–child observations had already led her to similar conclusions. She asserts that unresponsive and inconsistent mothering, or frequent harsh and negative maternal behavior, creates a condition wherein the toddler must devote inordinate inner resources to enlisting maternal contact and maintaining the mother–child connection, limiting the available neutralized energy that is needed for the progression of ego and early superego capacities.

The mother's affective availability rests on her own self-regulatory resources, which mitigate inevitable aggressive and sadistic responses to the toddler's hostility and ambivalence. Her capacity for emotional survival creates the security and continuity that the child requires in order to internalize stable object representations and build inner regulatory structures (Blum, 2004; Mahler, Pine, & Bergman, 1975; Sugarman, 2003; Winnicott, 1971). As Schaefer (1960) suggests, "how right or conflict-free the parent feels in his role of moral guide" is a key factor in the effective transmission of parental values and standards (p. 184). Maternal verbal communication, validation of the child's emotional experience, and promotion of coping mechanisms (e.g., shifting attention away from negative stimulation), in the face of toddler resistance and defiance, are empirically linked to the child's later acquisition of verbal negotiation and perspective-taking skills. Moreover, punitive and angry parental reactions are associated with an increase in the tendency toward negative arousal (Laible & Thompson, 2002; Spinrad et al., 2007).

The Role of Toilet Training

Although toilet training is one of myriad areas of parent socialization, its position in the toddler's mental life is unique, encompassing the entire range of developmental tasks such as separation–individuation, bodily awareness, self-control, identification with parental behavioral expectations, and acceptance of reality. Moreover, the initiation of the toileting process marks a turning point in the "bodily mother-child matrix" (Furman, 1996), as the parent's exclusive responsibility for the toddler's physical care is partially relinquished to the child (A. Freud, 1965). The child's gradual achievement of sphincter control represents a manifestation of early morality and self-regulation, reinforces self–other and inner–outer boundaries, and supports the sense of autonomy (Jacobson, 1954). Consolidation of anal phase defenses and identifications (e.g., reaction formations, internalization of parental standards for cleanliness, identification with the parent–aggressor), along with shared parent–toddler pride in the achievement of a major milestone, create a foundation for the child's continuing evolution toward cooperation, self-control, and independent functioning (Bach, 2002; Edgecumbe, 1978; A. Freud, 1965; Furman, 1996; Sandler & Freud, 1983; Yorke, 1982). The emergence of such anal themes as control, withholding, and dominance buffet the parent–child relationship, potentially evoking intense reactions from both individuals and creating a mutual environment of at least transient conflict. The mother's unconscious reluctance to yield possession of the toddler's body, feelings of loss that accompany the child's independence, and unresolved anal conflicts from her past may lead to excessive maternal anger, disgust, or fastidiousness over the child's attempts at self-management, or to premature emotional abandonment of the toddler (Furman, 1992, 1996). At the same time, the child's normative resistances, provocations, and teasing are potentially exacerbated by the mother's reactivity and disapproval. Specific anal-phase anxieties, which include increased awareness of genital-area sensations and concomitant fears of genital injury, as well as fantasies about the loss of precious bodily products, may further intensify the toddler's negative behavior. Unilateral, forceful maternal approaches to the toddler's body can exacerbate the child's aggressive urges, prolong the dyad's power struggles, and contribute to enduring anal trends, such as contrariness, pseudo-compliance, or interpersonal dominance. Furman (1992) distinguishes between "toilet training," wherein the parent imposes demands for the toddler's compliance, and "toilet mastery," a process that recruits the child's verbal and emotional capacities, encourages positive identifications with the parents, and fosters the child's autonomous strivings.

Cognitive Development

The toddler's cognitive achievements, typically seen as marking entry into the *preoperational phase* of intellectual development, include a proliferation of symbolic functions such as the acquisition of object permanence, the grasp of a categorical self-concept, a spurt in vocabulary and word combinations, and basic means–end problem solving (Bloom, 1993; Courage & Howe, 2002; Piaget, 1962a,b). Deferred imitation, a dominant mode of toddler–parent identification and a key forerunner to superego formation, is a defining behavior of this period, signaling the child's increasing capacity to employ mental representations rather than sensorimotor manipulation (Piaget, 1962b). Early forms of pretense, such as simple self-directed and mother-directed play, emerge between the first and second year of life, followed by more complex play scenarios that typically re-create familiar events (McCune, 1995). These various intellectual achievements significantly expand the toddler's capacity for self-regulation: The maternal presence can be evoked through memories, words, images, imitations, and pretense (Blum, 2004).

Nonetheless, the toddler's thinking is highly egocentric. Thought and action are poorly differentiated, and the child's mental contents, including wishes, fantasies, and dreams, are experienced as literal (Fonagy & Target, 1996). An exception to this is pretend play, which the toddler grasps as distinct from reality. Indeed, the infant's ability to discern marked affects in the mother suggests that pretense may reflect an innate human capacity (Emde, Kubicek, & Oppenheim, 1997). Naïve cognition powerfully shapes the toddler's fears about bodily intactness, manifested in age-typical phobias of such common phenomena as popped balloons or bathroom drains, and exacerbates anxiety about genital injury. Parental disapproval and punitive reactions are magnified by the child's fantasies of concrete dangers and threats. The toddler's confused "theories" about conception and birth, often conflated with digestive and eliminatory processes, lead to fantasies about the ubiquitous potential for pregnancy and raise concerns about the inherent destructiveness of defecation. External events, such as illness, injury, divorce, or sibling birth are potentially traumatic because of the toddler's egocentric interpretations (e.g., see Mitchell's 2006 description of the young child's experience of sibling birth). Moreover, although toddlers achieve a basic level of self–other mental differentiation, realizing that their desires do not always align with the mother's, meaningful links between behavior and mental states are not fully attained until the next phase of development. Fonagy and Target (1996) suggest that the gradual integration of the child's dual modes of thinking, that is, pretense (in which ideas are experienced as representations, but their correspondence with reality is not examined) and *psychic equivalence* (in which personal perception equals reality), is not achieved until around four years of age, at which point reality-testing is more firmly established and the child acquires a theory of mind (more fully explained in chapter 4).

Mother–child communication is fundamentally re-shaped during the toddler phase. Language increasingly functions as a major tool for sharing affective experience, transmitting cultural expectations, and achieving emotional self-regulation (Bloom, 1993; Parlade & Iverson, 2011; Rhee et al., 2013; Stern, 1985). At the end of infancy, an expressive vocabulary of three or four words is typical; by the age of two, many children have access to several hundred words and actively combine these into meaningful phrases, whereas oral comprehension is even more extensive (Bloom, 1993). As toddlers acquire mental state words (those signifying thoughts, desires, etc.) they are increasingly able to reflect on the self and share meanings with the parent (Bretherton & Beeghly, 1982; Courage & Howe, 2002). The child's acquisition of a mental state vocabulary is closely linked to the mother's capacity to mediate the toddler's experience through language and to function as an "emotional narrator" who interprets the toddler's experience (Harpez-Rotem & Bergman, 2006, p. 175). An expanding range of semantic comprehension facilitates socialization and self-control. The child grasps verbal prohibitions, using self-speech to reinforce the parental voice of authority and achieve self-direction during the parent's absence. Moreover, words and private monologues serve as transitional phenomena and self-soothing mechanisms during times of separation (Nelson, 1989). Indeed, one pair of authors has commented that "the road to object constancy is paved with language" (Blum & Blum, 1990, p. 545), noting that verbal capacities facilitate the child's progression to the next phase of development.

Summary

The toddler phase, roughly encompassing the years between the first and third birthdays, is marked by a vastly increased awareness of the self and the external world. Upright mobility, along with underlying cognitive and linguistic advances contribute to the child's realization of personal separateness and vulnerability, creating renewed fears of object loss and demands for maternal contact; competing desires for autonomy and security lead to the ambivalent, contradictory behaviors that are the hallmark of the rapprochement period. The toddler begins to internalize parental standards of behavior. Responsibility for bodily functions and self-control is gradually shifted from the mother to the child, most notably within the context of toilet training. Forerunners of superego development, such as the wished-for self-image, are manifest in the toddler's active imitations and identifications with parental actions. The parent's capacity to remain constant and warmly available, in the face of the toddler's ambivalence and negativity, facilitates the acquisition of stable, internalized object representations and loving self-feelings. Libidinal object constancy fosters resolution of the rapprochement dilemma and facilitates entry into the oedipal phase of development.

Hallmarks of the toddler phase include the following:

- At around 15 to 18 months, a new level of self-awareness and an increased sense of separateness emerges, leading to a period of separation anxiety and renewed desire for contact with the parent. Contradictory behaviors and moodiness reflect the toddler's competing desires for autononomy and intimacy.
- Vastly expanded symbolic capacities, including language and imitation, contribute to the parents' expectations for bodily and emotional self-control. The processes of socialization, such as toilet training, are often initiated at between two and three years of age. The toddler is increasingly aware of parental prohibitions and approval, and self-conscious,

self-evaluative emotions (e.g., pride and shame) accompany the child's behaviors.

· Emerging language and play, along with more stable inner representations of relationships, equip the toddler with greatly enhanced emotional self-regulatory capacities.

References

Bach, S. (2002). Sadomasochism in clinical practice and everyday life. *Journal of Clinical Psychoanalysis, 11*, 225–235.

Bergman, A., & Harpaz-Rotem, I. (2004). Revisiting rapprochement in the light of contemporary developmental theories. *Journal of the American Psychoanalytic Association, 52*, 555–570.

Bloom, L. (1993). *The Transition from Infancy to Language: Acquiring the Power of Expression.* New York: Cambridge University Press.

Blos, P. (1967). The second individuation process of adolescence. *Psychoanalytic Study of the Child, 22*, 162–186.

Blum, H. P. (2004). Separation-individuation theory and attachment theory. *Journal of the American Psychoanalytic Association, 52*, 535–553.

Blum, E. J. & Blum, H. P. (1990). The development of autonomy and superego precursors. *International Journal of Psychoanalysis, 71*, 585–595.

Bretherton, I. & Beeghly, M. (1982). Talking about internal states: the acquisition of an explicit theory of mind. *Developmental Psychology, 18*, 906–921.

Buchsbaum, H. K. & Emde, R. N. (1990). Play narratives in 36-month-old children: early moral development and family relations. *Psychoanalytic Study of the Child, 45*, 129–155.

Courage, M. L. & Howe, M. L. (2002). From infancy to childhood: the dynamics of cognitive change in the second year of life. *Psychology Bulletin, 128*, 250–277.

DeMarneffe, D. (1997). Bodies and words: a study of young children's genital and gender knowledge. *Gender and Psychoanalysis, 2*, 3–33.

Dix, T., Stewart, A. D., Gershoff, E. T., & Day, W. H. (2007). Autonomy and children's reactions to being controlled: evidence that both compliance and defiance may be positive markers in early development. *Child Development, 78*, 1204–1221.

Edgecumbe, R. (1978). The psychoanalytic view of the development of encopresis. *Bulletin of the Anna Freud Centre, 1*, 57–61.

Emde, R. N., Biringen, Z., Clyman, R. B., & Oppenheim, D. (1991). The moral self of infancy: affective core and procedural knowledge. *Developmental Review, 11*, 251–270.

Emde, R. N., Johnson, W. F., & Easterbrooks, M. A. (1987). The do's and don'ts of early moral development: psychoanalytic tradition and current research. In J. Kagan & S. Lamb (Eds.), *The Emergence of Morality in Young Children* (pp. 245–276). Chicago: Chicago University Press.

Emde, R. N., Kubicek, L., & Oppenheim, D. (1997). Imaginative reality observed during early language. *International Journal of Psychoanalysis, 78*, 115–133.

Ferenczi, S. (1925). Psycho-analysis of sexual habits. In *Further Contributions to the Theory and Technique of Psycho-analysis, 1950* (pp. 259–297). London: Hogarth Press.

Fonagy, P., Target, M. (1996). Playing with reality: I. Theory of mind and the normal development of psychic reality. *International Journal of Psychoanalysis, 77*, 217–233.

Freud, A. (1936). *The Ego and the Mechanisms of Defense.* New York: International University Press.

Freud, A. (1965). *Normality and Pathology in Childhood: Assessments of Development.* New York: International University Press.

Freud, S. (1917). On transformations of instinct as exemplified in anal erotism. In J. Strachey (Ed. & Trans.), *The Standard Edition of the Complete Works of Sigmund Freud* (Vol. 17). London: Hogarth Press.

Furman, E. (1992). *Toddlers and Their Mothers.* Madison, CT: International University Press.

Furman, E. (1996). On motherhood. *Journal of American Psychoanalytic Association, 44S*, 429–447.

Gergely, G. (2000). Repproaching Mahler: new perspectives on normal autism, symbiosis splitting and libidinal object constancy from cognitive developmental theory. *Journal of the American Psychoanalytic Association, 48*, 1197–1228.

Gilmore, K. (1998). Cloacal anxiety in female development. *Journal of the American Psychoanalytic Association, 46*, 443–470.

Greenacre, P. (1957). The childhood of the artist—libidinal phase development and giftedness. *Psychoanalytic Study of the Child, 12*, 47–72.

Harpez-Rotem, I. & Bergman, A. (2006). On an evolving theory of attachment: rapprochement—theory of a developing mind. *Psychoanalytic Study of the Child, 61*, 170–189.

Holder, A. (1982). Preoedipal contributions to the formation of the superego. *Psychoanalytic Study of the Child, 37,* 245–272.

Jacobson, E. (1954). The self and the object world—vicissitudes of their infantile cathexes and their influence on ideational and affective development. *Psychoanalytic Study of the Child, 9,* 75–127.

Kennedy, H. & Yorke, C. (1982). Steps from outer to inner conflict viewed as superego precursors. *Psychoanalytic Study of the Child, 37,* 221–228.

Kochansksa, G., Aksan, N., Knaack, A., & Rhines, H. (2004). Maternal parenting and children's conscience: early security as moderator. *Child Development, 75,* 1229–1242.

Kochanska, G., Koenig, S. L., Barry, R. A., Kim, S., & Yoon, J. E. (2010). Children's conscience during toddler and preschool years, moral self, and a competent, adaptive developmental trajectory. *Developmental Psychology, 46,* 1320–1332.

Laible, D. J., Panfile, T., & Makariev, D. (2008). The quality and frequency of mother-toddler conflict: links with attachment and temperament. *Child Development, 79,* 426–443.

Laible, D. J. & Thompson, R. A. (2002). Mother-child conflict in the toddler years: lessons in emotional, morality and relationships. *Child Development, 73,* 1187–1203.

Lewis, M. & Brooks-Gunn, J. (1979). Toward a theory of social cognition: the development of the self. *New Directions for Child Development, 4,* 1–20.

Lyons-Ruth, K. (1991). Rapprochement or approchement: Mahler's theory reconsidered from the vantage point of recent research on early attachment relationships. *Psychoanalytic Psychology, 8,* 1–23.

Mahler, M. (1963). Thoughts about development and individuation. *Psychoanalytic Study of the Child, 18,* 307–324.

Mahler, M. (1972). Rapprochement subphase of the separation-individuation process. *Psychoanalytic Quarterly, 41,* 487–506.

Mahler, M., Pine, F., & Bergman, A. (1975). *The Psychological Birth of the Human Infant.* New York: Basic Books.

Mahler, M. S., & McDevitt, J. B. (1968). Observations on adaptation and defense in statu nascendi developmental precursors in the first two years of life. *Psychoanalytic Quarterly, 37,* 1–21.

Masterson, J. F., & Rinsley, D. B. (1975). The borderline syndrome: the role of the mother in the genesis and psychic structure of the borderline personality. *International Journal of Psychoanalysis, 56,* 163–177.

Martin, C. L., & Ruble, D. (2004). Children's search for gender cues. *Current Directions in Psychological Science, 13,* 67–70.

McCune, L. (1995). A normative study of representational play at the transition to language. *Developmental Psychology, 31,* 198–206.

McDevitt, J. (1975). Separation-individuation and object constancy. *Journal of the American Psychoanalytic Association, 23,* 712–742.

Meissner, W. W. (2009). The genesis of the self II: progression from rapprochement to adolescence. *Psychoanalytic Review, 96,* 261–295.

Milrod, D. (1982). The wished-for self-image. *Psychoanalytic Study of the Child, 37,* 95–120.

Milrod, D. (2002). The superego: its formation, structure and functioning. *Psychoanalytic Study of the Child, 57,* 131–148.

Mitchell, J. (2006). From infant to child: the sibling trauma, the rite de passage and the construction of the "other" in the social group. *Fort Da, 12,* 35–49.

Nelson, K. (1989). *Narratives from the Crib.* MA: Harvard University Press.

Olesker, W. (1998). Female genital anxieties: views from the nursery and the couch. *Psychoanalytic Quarterly, 61,* 331–351.

Parlade, M. V. & Iverson, J. M. (2011). The interplay between language, gesture and affect during communicative transition: a dynamic systems approach. *Developmental Psychology, 47,* 820–833.

Piaget, J. (1952). *The Origins of Intelligence in Children.* New York: International University Press.

Piaget, J. (1962a). *Language and Thought of the Child.* London: Routledge Press.

Piaget, J. (1962b). *Play, Dreams and Imitation in Childhood.* New York: Norton.

Rhee, S. H., Boeldt, D. L., Friedman, N. P., Corley, C. P., Hewitt, J. K., Young, S. E., et al. (2013). The role of language in concern and disregard for others in the 1st years of life. *Developmental Psychology, 49,* 197–214.

Sandler, J. (1960). On the concept of superego. *Psychoanalytic Study of the Child, 15,* 128–162.

Sandler, J. & Freud, A. (1983). Discussions in the Hampstead Index on "The ego and the mechanisms of defence." X. Identification with the aggressor. *Bulletin of the Anna Freud Centre, 6,* 247–275.

Schafer, R. (1960). The loving and beloved superego in Freud's structural theory. *Psychoanalytic Study of the Child, 15,* 163–188.

Senet, N. V. (2004). A study of preschool children's linking of genitals and gender. *Psychoanalytic Quarterly, 73*, 291–334.

Shengold, L. (1985). Defensive anality and anal narcissism. *International Journal of Psychoanalysis, 66*, 47–73.

Spinrad, T., Eisenberg, N., Gaertner, B., Popp, T., Smith, C. L., Kupfer, A., et al. (2007). Relationship of maternal socialization and toddler's effortful control to children's adjustment and social competence. *Developmental Psychology, 43*, 1170–1186.

Spitz, R. A. (1957). *No and Yes: On the Genesis of Human Communication.* New York: International University Press.

Stern, D. N. (1985). *The Interpersonal World of the Infant: A View from Psychoanalysis and Developmental Psychology.* New York: Basic Books.

Stipek, D. J., Gralinski, J. H., & Koop, C. B. (1990). Self-conscious development in the toddler years. *Developmental Psychology, 26*, 972–977.

Sugarman, A. (2003). Dimensions of the child analyst's role as a developmental object: affect regulation and limit setting. *Psychoanalytic Study of the Child, 58*, 189–218.

Vaish, A., Missana, M., & Tomasello, M. (2011). Three year old children intervene in third party moral transgressions. *British Journal of Developmental Psychology, 29*, 124–130.

Winnicott, D. W. (1971). *Playing and Reality.* London: Tavistock Publications.

Yorke, C. (1982). The development of the sense of shame. *Psychoanalytic Study of the Child, 45*, 377–409.

4

The Oedipal Phase and the Oedipal Complex: Developmental Advances and Theoretical Considerations

Overview

"It has justly been said that the Oedipus complex is the nuclear complex of the neuroses, and constitutes the essential part of their content. It represents the peak of infantile sexuality, which, through its after-effects, exercises a decisive influence on the sexuality of adults. Every new arrival on this planet is faced by the task of mastering the Oedipus complex; anyone who fails to do so falls a victim to neurosis. With the progress of psycho-analytic studies the importance of the Oedipus complex has become more and more clearly evident; its recognition has become the shibboleth that distinguishes the adherents of psycho-analysis from its opponents."

(FREUD, 1905/1953 [footnote added 1920], p. 226)

This chapter examines the oedipal phase and its associated complex, which, until very recently, have been widely considered the centerpiece of psychoanalytic theorizing (Simon, 1991). Although the phase and the complex are closely and substantively linked in Freud's original formulation (the phase generating the complex), they represent significantly different levels of abstraction within psychological thinking. One is a developmental period and the other is an experience of intense emotions toward central figures that leaves a persistent, structured, unconscious intrapsychic constellation in the mind (Loewald, 1970). Both phase and complex are powerfully shaped by the individual child's own unique repertoire of emerging capacities and physiological maturation, his or her basic endowment, caretaking environment, and prior experience. Despite remarkable diversity among individuals in this phase and variations of the mental construct as it is inferred from psychoanalytic data, oedipal children are recognizable as similar, and some variant of the oedipal complex is arguably observable in everyone. Even if the trends in divorce rate, composition of families, and reproductive methodologies alter the basic realties of childhood that form the matrix of oedipal experience, the developmental transformation will likely continue to be recognizable.

The oedipal phase and complex stand out among Freud's major insights, embedded in his then-revolutionary discovery of infantile sexuality and theory of psychosexual development. We continue to find enormous clinical value in these ideas. The oedipal phase marks an advance in mental development that reverberates in subsequent personality transformations. However, we no longer share many of Freud's premises and are influenced by a very different cultural zeitgeist. Attitudes toward female development are a case in point. Advances in our understanding over the last century, both in regard to theory and developmental research, have corrected many of Freud's ideas. In what follows we select from among the innumerable contributions in the literature that continue to serve the clinician; describe the array of emerging capacities that characterize this phase; address the nature of the child's intense desires and conflicts; present a modern view of the phase and the significance of the complex in regard to pathogenesis; reformulate the formation of the superego; and describe variations in oedipal configurations and their impact on mental development.

Early Views

As the opening quotation indicates, Freud posited that the complex, arising in the context of the child's dawning awareness of family roles and relationships and his or her heightened, biologically driven focus on the genital (the phallic phase of psychosexual development), forms the foundation for the mental organization of the adult. Moreover, the child's solution to the conflicts of this phase determines health or neurosis in later life. Experiencing and then "mastering" the oedipal complex is the task that occupies the child in the years between toddlerhood and latency, roughly three to six years old, known as "the oedipal" or "genital" phase. In Freud's original formulation of psychosexual development, the genital phase is both a culmination and integration of prior forms of erogenous excitation. The leading zone is now the genital, and pregenital sources of excitation (oral and anal), and their associated component instincts are subordinated to genital pleasure.

Because Freud believed that the young child is ignorant of the anatomical basis of sex differences and knows only one genital (the phallus), he suggested that before the genital oedipal phase in which the adult sexual pattern is set, there is a prodromal phallic phase (Freud, 1923), in which infantile misperceptions rule and interest in displaying the genital or the whole body for the admiration of beloved others is prominent. Subsequent observers within the ego psychological tradition have offered elaborations or revisions of these ideas. Observers at the Hampstead Clinic suggested that there is a phallic-narcissistic phase preceding the full triadic flowering of the oedipal complex (Edgcumbe & Burgner, 1975). The primary focus on the phallus was hypothesized to evolve in advance of object relations, thus in a dyadic context that is not yet matched by object relational advances toward triadic relationships. In this subphase, both the boy and girl seek the admiration and exclusive interest of the desired parent. They both wish to exhibit and are deeply interested in looking. For the boy this is manifested in exhibitionism regarding his penis, whereas the girl enjoys a display of her whole body. Both are curious and eager to pursue sexual researches by peeking at intimate encounters (scoptophilia), establishing the central importance of the *primal scene* (see glossary) as a paradigm of erotic excitement, exclusion, and narcissistic mortification. The phallic–narcissistic phase predates the true genital phase, which gradually emerges in the context of fully established recognition of sexual differences, with associated castration anxiety in the boy and narcissistic deflation in the girl.

In Freud's formulation, the role of castration anxiety and penis envy are distinguishing features in the oedipal passage of the two sexes. For boys, the threat of castration ushers in the repression of oedipal ambitions and identification with the father. In contrast, for girls the realization of their "already castrated" condition sets their oedipal dynamic in motion, as they turn in disappointment from their mothers to their fathers and seek consolation in the idea of obtaining a baby. Subsequent observational research specifically in regard to the girl's development supported a more complex picture with variations in the girl's progression into the oedipal complex. She can be propelled there by disappointment that her mother failed to provide an organ comparable to the boys, she can enter into the complex through a primary maternal desire for a baby, or by a combination of ambivalence toward her mother, castration fears, and her interest in her father as an object of desire (Parens, 1990).

Freud postulated that the waning of the oedipus complex and the "formation" of the superego follows different courses for the boy and the girl. The boy's renunciation of oedipal desires is a direct result of the newly discovered vulnerability of his treasured organ, his growing disillusionment in regard to his infantile grandiosity, and his profound ambivalent conflicts in regard to his parents who are now viewed as rivals or rejecters; the superego forms as an internal support and a source of self-esteem. The boy regains a sense of goodness and safety by virtue of internalizing his father's guiding voice and values, identifying with his manly features, and accepting the idea that he must wait to assume his father's place. For the girl, her "moral efforts are exhausted by her acceptance of castration" (Jacobson, 1976, p. 534) and her phallic narcissism gives way to feelings of inferiority. Her turn to her father substitutes object love for the self-contained love of an internalized voice. Superego function is transferred to the father and only partially internalized. Thus in classical Freudian theory, differences in superego development are closely tied to the biological sex of the child. The boy is hastened into oedipal resolution and superego consolidation by castration anxiety, whereas the girl's recognition of genital differences shifts her focus to the father but provides no incentive to renounce oedipal desire or assume a self-policing function.

Early conceptualizations certainly emphasize the central importance of psychosexual development, but nonetheless contain inherent potential for complexity and a discernible multisystemic interface. Freud's formulation recognizes that the oedipal situation is characterized by multiplicity. There is the original "positive" formation and the inevitable "negative" configuration, wherein the same-sex parent is favored and the opposite-sex parent is the rival. The child's engagement in the oedipal triangle of love, desire, competition, and hate with parents in itself reflects a step forward in his or her object relations and emotional repertoire. The presumed optimal resolution—the foregoing of the desired parent and identification with the rival—requires a further advance in object relations and the defensive repertoire, such that repression becomes the primary mechanism of defense in contrast to the use of splitting. The child's specific triangular force field is repressed, facilitating enhanced identification with the rival parent, consolidation of sexual and gender identity, access to the mental energy required for learning, and the formation of the superego. The child enters into the "adult world" and "moral order" (Loewald, 1985). These achievements herald the libidinally quiescent period of latency. They influence later appetites for learning, narcissistic equilibrium, conscience, ambition, sexual identity, sexual orientation, goals, and values.

Modern Perspectives on the Oedipus

The hegemony of the oedipal complex, the oedipal phase, and the achievement of "oedipal-level" development in psychoanalytic theorizing has persisted for decades. Objections to its traditional formulation and emphasis emerged from a range of thinkers, including feminist writers, queer theorists, self-psychologists, and postmodern relationalists. Contemporary pluralism in and of itself has eroded its centrality, and the transformations in today's nuclear family have introduced a radically altered context for the oedipal phase of development (Corbett, 2001; Heineman, 2004). In what follows, we selectively address some of these challenges to the Oedipus and the questions they raise. Are the unconscious fantasies that derive from the oedipal complex as timeless and enduring as they once seemed? Is the experience of the oedipal triangle critical for emotional depth and complexity, morality, and interpersonal maturity? Is the oedipal constellation as deeply woven into the human experience and human mental legacy as Freud and his followers believe? We also highlight the profound psychological advances that occur during this phase, especially the emergence of ego capacities that revolutionize the child's relationship to the world at large, brilliantly captured by, but also independent of, the oedipal metaphor. Finally, we address the value of the oedipal complex's continued prominence in psychoanalytic thinking.

The Developmental Capacities of the Oedipal Phase

Despite diverse perspectives about its ultimate legacy in adult mental life, the oedipal phase is universally viewed as a watershed period in the child's psychological development. A proliferation of semiotic functions—language, imaginative fantasy, play, and *mentalization*—transforms the egocentric perspective of the toddler, leading to sharper distinctions between inner and outer experience and a dawning awareness of individuals' subjectivities. These newly emergent, interconnected capacities vastly increase the child's potential for relational and emotional complexity, while enhancing cognitive control and emotional self-regulation. Together, they support the emergence of new mental organizations that are foundational for forward development, including triadic relationships, complex fantasy, and superego formation.

Traditional psychoanalytic theory has viewed the child's acquisition of increasingly stable, internalized object representations and self–other differentiation as key developmental tasks of early childhood. Libidinal object constancy (Mahler, 1971; Mahler, Pine, & Bergman, 1975), a unified, internalized relationship capable of retaining its qualities in the face of emotional upheaval, has been seen as a prerequisite for the full flowering and consolidation of the oedipal complex (Blum, 2010). However, contemporary concepts such as mentalization and emotional self-regulation have largely supplanted these ideas. We nonetheless believe that certain basic psychoanalytic formulations, such as libidinal object constancy, retain enormous relevance and meaningfully capture the child's struggle with heightened sexual and aggressive urges that fuel the oedipal drama. Certainly, the emphasis that Mahler and others place on the mother's ongoing availability and consistency in the face of the child's ambivalence is echoed by more current research examining the maternal role in fostering mentalization, conscience, and emotional self-control. The gradual shift toward greater self–other differentiation (both in the sense of separate bodies and individual, subjective minds) and the overall arc of development from external to more fully internalized conflicts and toward increasingly reliable inner structures for self-regulation are noted by both psychoanalytic and empirical writers (Bretherton, 1990; Fonagy & Target, 1996; Harris, De Rosnay, & Pons, 2005; Kochanska, Coy, & Murray, 2001; Laible & Thompson, 2000; Mahler, Pine, & Bergman, 1975). At the same time, empirically based work offers distinctive and heretofore unrealized clarifications of the oedipal child's deepening capacity for intersubjectivity and of the ongoing, dyadic processes from which stable emotional and moral functioning ultimately emerges. The following sections briefly review psychoanalytic and empirical thinking about the developmental tasks of the oedipal phase.

Language Development

An explosion of linguistic capacities is inextricably linked to the oedipal child's development of fantasy and play, the acquisition of mental state knowledge and complex relationships, the enhancement of self-regulation and control, and the emergence of higher-level logic and problem-solving abilities. Unlike the toddler, whose speech is closely tied to immediate perceptual experience, the preschool child begins to talk and think about abstractions, using a vastly increased lexicon, more complicated syntax, a facility with past and future tense, and an expanding grasp of ideas. The growing sophistication in the use of language facilitates self-reflection and introduces implicitly grasped experience into the child's conscious awareness. A major influence is discourse with significant others, which instantiates secondary representations of meaningful events and provides opportunities to interpret interpersonal situations (Laible & Song, 2006; Nelson, 1996).

Private, self-directed talk (labeled "egocentric speech" by Piaget [1926]) often accompanies the young child's play and problem-solving activities. In contrast to the toddler's reliance on wishful self-images, the oedipal child increasingly uses verbal self-directives to retain and consolidate the parents' vocalized standards, manage emotional arousal, delay gratification, and inhibit urges (Migden, 1998; Winsler, 2003). Moreover, the internalized moral "voice" of the parent acquires deeper meaning as the child begins to grasp such verbal abstractions as goodness and kindness and to endow these with increased status and desirability. Classic, beloved narratives and fairy tales, now within the child's linguistic reach, serve as additional reinforcement for moral messages (Bettelheim, 1975). Indeed, language capacities are empirically linked to the child's acquisition of conscience and behavioral self-control and are foundational to the preschooler's ability to self-initiate regulatory strategies (Cole, Armstrong, & Pemberton, 2010; Laible & Thompson, 2000; Peterson et al., 2013).

Furthermore, language serves key functions in deepening the young child's knowledge about mental states. At around the age of two, verbal expressions of desire (e.g., "I want") emerge, soon followed by statements about beliefs ("I think") (Ruffman, Slade, & Crowe, 2002). As linguistic use and comprehension increase, the child's inevitable exposure to others' accounts of events and their differing perspectives on reality is instrumental in diminishing egocentricity and acquiring the gradual realization that one's own internal experience is subjective (Piaget, 1926). Nelson (1996) observes that "it is only through language that children can be sure that someone else's experience of a situation is different from their own" (p. 340). Exposure to maternal dialogue that contains affectively laden material and psychological themes is linked to the development of mental state knowledge and moral reasoning (Carlson, Mandell, & Williams, 2004; Harris, de Rosnay, & Pons, 2005). The emotionally available mother, through her verbal elaborations of feeling states, promotes the preschool child's curiosity about and exploration of the mind in much the same way as, at an earlier age, she fostered her infant's secure investigation of the physical surround (Oppenheim, Koren-Karie, & Sagi-Schwartz, 2007).

The emergence of narrative capacities and narrative-based autobiographical memories profoundly alters the child's sense of self, capacity to self-regulate and ability to make and share meaning. Shortly before the third birthday, children begin to employ basic story structure for recounting events. Initially, narrative-creation is heavily scaffolded by the parent (Haden, Haine, & Fivush, 1997). Narrative-making is closely linked to the management of internal states: personal or literary stories serve to organize and make sense of intense feelings and wishes (Emde, Kubicek, & Oppenheim, 1997; Knight, 2003). The vivid characters, plots, and highly moralistic themes of timeless fairy tales (such as Cinderella or Sleeping Beauty) are particularly suited to the oedipal child's interior struggles over sexual and aggressive urges (Bettelheim, 1975). Ultimately, mental life is organized around powerful, enduring self-narratives that are intimately connected to affective states and self-feelings (Ginot, 2012; Nelson, 1996). In an elucidation of the cognitive, emotional, and somatic origins of dysregulated states, Ginot (2012) suggests that narratives "become the cognitive expression of affective dysregulation, containing within them past interactions, emotional memories, defenses and distorted conclusions, all triggered by emotional stresses activating implicit schemas" (p. 60). Indeed, for children and adults alike, maintaining narrative coherence in the face of emotionally laden experience is viewed as a hallmark of secure attachment (Main, 2000).

Imaginary Play

The emergence of abstract language, narrative competence and mentalization equips the oedipal child for exponentially increased fantasy potential, most vividly depicted in pretend (or symbolic) play. Imagination serves as a synthesizing ego function, contributing significantly to the expansion of the child's internal object world and emotional self-regulatory resources. It promotes trial thought and action, strengthens identifications, and enables the child to "tolerate multiple, often conflicting views of the object relational world" (Mayes & Cohen, 1992, p. 26). In contrast to the toddler's play, which tends toward simple recreations of familiar events, the three- and four-year-old child begins to initiate unique, creative characters and storylines of increasing complexity. Vygotsky (1978) hypothesized symbolic play as a potential zone of proximal development wherein children demonstrate heightened availability to novel cognition. In his view, the separation of object and referent, a key aspect of pretense, contributes to the child's growing capacity for abstract thinking. Contemporary research largely supports the notion of play as a unique state in which the child's cognition appears advanced beyond age expectations. For example, the three-year-old child who has not yet attained reliable theory of mind and who is only beginning to differentiate internal experience (e.g., dreams, wishes) from external events evidences no confusion over the distinction between pretend play and reality, and regularly attributes beliefs and desires to imaginary characters (Emde, Kubicek, & Oppenheim, 1997; Mayes & Cohen, 1996).

The capacity for pretense appears early in infancy, with the baby's ability to distinguish between the mother's real and marked affects (Gergely, 2000). Symbolic play, wherein one concrete object substitutes for another, emerges early in the second year of life. More abstract symbolic replacements and simple fantasy play are evident before the age of three years, although sustained, complex, and creative pretense develops after the third birthday (Fein, 1981). By the age of four, most children engage extensively in collaborative fantasy play with peers. The shift to sociodramatic play requires

complex cognitive and linguistic capacities, such as verbal negotiation about storylines, role assignments, and agreement on the symbolic transformation of available objects (Howe et al., 2005).
A recent meta-review of empirical studies failed to confirm
causal links between play and other cognitive, emotional, and social
functions (Lillard et al., 2013), but the correlation between play
and good developmental outcome has been universally recognized.
Psychoanalysts have long privileged play as a natural, uniquely revelatory, and growth-promoting function of childhood that serves as
a dominant mode of intersubjective sharing and communication,
converts passive into active experience, provides opportunities for
trying on new roles and identifications, allows for the expression
and transformation of wishes and impulses in a nonconsequential
setting, and promotes adaptive solutions to both conscious and
unconscious conflicts (Cohen et al., 1987; Freud, 1920; Neubauer,
1987; Gilmore, 2005, 2011; Mayes & Cohen, 1992). The empirical approach emphasizes the role of solitary and peer play in the
child's practice and mastery of newfound cognitive, linguistic, and
problem-solving skills as well as in promoting theory of mind and
social collaboration (Howe et al, 2005; Lyons-Ruth, 2006; Marans
et al., 1991). Other forms of playful fantasy, such as imaginary
friends and characters also emerge during the preschool period
and are similarly linked to the development of social and emotional
competence (Meyer & Tuber, 1989).

Although pretense often continues in some form throughout
the duration of childhood, the oedipal phase is peak season for the
child's passionate absorption in pretend activities (Gilmore, 2011;
Singer & Singer, 1992). The process of imaginary play and its accompanying fantasy themes—typically domestic, romantic, or adven-
turous—are uniquely suited to the externalization and displacement
of the oedipal child's heightened state of conflict and excitation.
Playing Mommy, princess, or hero dramatically depicts oedipal dramas, giving free reign to disguised urges while connecting these
to organized, meaningful narratives. Imaginary transformation
of the child into a wished-for persona assuages intense desire for
adult power and status and consolidates identification with adult

standards and perceived gender qualities. Moreover, the "pretense mode" of the playing state, in which reality concerns are safely suspended, helps sharpen the distinction between interior subjectivity and the external world; imaginary play promotes the oedipal child's capacity to reflect on affective states, a key function of mentalization intimately connected to the use of psychological resources (e.g., fantasy and reflection) rather than action-based solutions to emotional arousal (Fonagy & Target, 1996; Jurist, 2005).

Mentalization and Theory of Mind

Both psychoanalytic and developmental thinkers view the emergence of the young child's capacity to reflect on another's perspective and make meaning of people's behavior as benchmarks of psychological development. Within the empirical literature, the signature acquisition of a *theory of mind*, a network of concepts that governs how people interpret and predict human behavior, has been a focus of extensive inquiry. Theory of mind encompasses the notions that behavior and mental states are differentiated but linked, that beliefs drive not only people's actions but also their feelings, and that motivational beliefs may be false; it is generally consolidated by around four years of age (Mayes & Cohen, 1996). However, more subtle ramifications of theory of mind, such as the realization that people's manifest reactions can differ from feelings that are privately held, are grasped slightly later, at five or six years (Ruffman et al., 2002).

Psychoanalytic thinkers tend to focus on the related process of mentalization (Fonagy & Target, 1996), which refers to the capacity to understand one's own and others' minds. This development is inextricably linked to the child's affective sense of self and emerges within the context of the mother's emotional availability, particularly the marked and contingent reactions that promote the infant's representations of affect states. Mentalization can be disrupted by maltreatment or other traumatic events (Fonagy & Target, 1996; Weinberg, 2006). Such emphasis meaningfully distinguishes it from the more cognitive-based theory of mind concept, and connects mentalization closely with attachment theory, as well as the psychoanalytic writings of Winnicott and Bion. The acquisition of theory of mind and mentalization capacities supports reality testing, provides the child with a deeper and more abstract sense of self–other differentiation and human subjectivity, vastly enhances emotional self-regulation, and contributes to the growing capacity for triadic relationships.

A considerable body of research on theory of mind acquisition has yielded an orderly, sequential unfolding of capacities, culminating at around the age of four years, with individual differences in the rate of progress (Harris, De Rosnay, & Pons, 2005; Woolley & Wellman, 1993). Early forms of mental state knowledge and the capacity to share another's feelings and intentions emerge during infancy and are manifest through such mother–child interactions as joint attention and social referencing (see chapter 2). Toddlers begin to talk about mental states, referring to their own and others' emotions. By age three, children distinguish between mental and external events, and have rudimentary theories about how to predict people's actions (Wellman, Phillips, & Rodriguez, 2000). Moreover, in their pretend play, three-year-olds readily attribute differentiated desires and beliefs to their characters (Mayes & Cohen, 1996). However, some aspects of egocentricity remain. For example, although three-year-olds grasp the basic notion of subjective desires, they may have trouble with social reasoning that involves wishes that are in direct conflict with their own (Moll et al., 2013).

Historically, the empirical investigation into theory of mind has encompassed both appearance/reality tasks, which focus on physical properties, and false belief tasks, which involve social thinking. A classic perceptual task involves the following scenario. A youngster is visually confronted with an item that looks like a rock. Manual exploration, however, reveals the object's sponge-like qualities (Flavell, Flavell, & Green, 1983). Consistently, children younger than the age of four years fail to hold in mind and integrate these competing pieces of information. When asked to describe the object, four-year-olds correctly state that it looks like a rock but is or feels like a sponge, whereas younger children insist that it both looks like and is either a rock or sponge (Moll & Tomasello, 2012). False belief tasks pose social perspective-taking dilemmas. These are designed to elicit the child's realization that experience and knowledge are subjective, and that someone's behavior may be driven by incorrect beliefs. For example, the child is presented with the following story. While a girl is out of the room, someone moves her cookie from place A to place B. Will she search first in place A or place B when she returns? Before the age of four, children tend to have trouble differentiating their own knowledge from that of the story actor, and respond that she will initially look in place B (Wimmer & Perner, 1983).

Enhanced awareness of others' separate, subjective inner lives has far-reaching implications for oedipal phase functioning, as well as for subsequent childhood outcome. Acquisition of theory of mind is empirically linked to the emergence of empathy and prosocial behavior, social competence, self-control, and emotional self-regulation (Denhan et al., 2003; Fonagy & Target, 1996; Mayes & Cohen, 1996), all cornerstones for the formation of superego structure. Diminishing egocentricity, increased awareness of others' desires and needs, and the ability to differentiate these from personal wishes creates unprecedented availability for relationships beyond the dyad, and for triadic experience, but also lead to novel vulnerabilities, such as sharper feelings of exclusion, competition, and jealousy.

Differences between the Sexes, Gender Development, and the Superego

Emerging capacities allow the oedipal age child to experience self, family members, and family relationships with a new, often overwhelming level of intensity. The importance of sex and gender as potent identifiers, and the mystery and excitement of conception and sexual differences are enhanced in the mind of the oedipal child. Overall, the remarkable transformation of the passionate youngster embedded in a force-field of love, rivalry, hatred, and desire into the (at least superficially) becalmed school-oriented latency child requires the many cognitive and socio-emotional capacities described above. The simplified causality of Freud's early theorizing, attributing the structuralization of the superego and the move into latency to a castration threat, is no longer tenable. What remains remarkable is Freud's profoundly insightful observations about the importance of this developmental moment.

Freud's thinking about the differences between boys' and girls' development as they traverse the oedipal phase and move toward latency was undoubtedly skewed by his cultural zeitgeist. Even among his contemporaries, objections were raised in regard to his formulations about sex-linked superego differences and gender development in general. Today's thinkers from within and outside the Freudian tradition have further criticized or modified his ideas. In our opinion, delinking the multidimensional developmental gains crammed into this period from a singular psychosexual driver does much to liberate us from some of Freud's more outmoded assertions. Our perspective about boys' and girls' early development acknowledges the importance of the body and its role in mental development, but also recognizes the powerful messages and meanings that begin immediately, in response to the identification of the infant's sex at birth or before. Communications about gender (a psychological construct) begin in the earliest encounters and continue to accrue during each developmental stage. There is ample evidence that boys and girls are acquainted with the categorization of male and female well before the oedipal period and usually "know" what sex they are. There is also research data showing that meanings associated with such knowledge are not dependent on anatomical differentiation. Young children identify themselves and others correctly based on features such as hair length and outfit. Consolidation of the connection between biological sex and the anatomical genital becomes reliable only by 36 months (DeMarneffe, 1997). No doubt this timing reverberates with the many systems that are advancing toward a new level of complexity, including the cognitive capacities to comprehend and integrate these connections into the self-representation.

In the oedipal phase, the sex- and gender-related ideas and identifications take a central role in the highly fraught emotional drama
unfolding in the child's intimate relationships. Sexual identity and
gender identity thus contribute to the oedipal configuration but
also emerge from it transformed and enhanced as defining features
of the self. Castration fears and fantasies are indeed a part of the
oedipal experience insofar as the genital, gradually understood as
the crucial factor in sex assignment and appreciated as a source
of pleasure, takes on such importance. Bodily differences arouse
curiosity and comparison in boys and girls. Because young children value "more" and "fancy," it is not uncommon for girls to be
somewhat chagrinned by observations of boys' more conspicuous
external genital equipment, but they also value and enjoy their own
genital sensations and configuration, experience sex-specific anxieties (Bernstein, 1990; Gilmore, 1998; Mayer, 1985; Olesker, 1998),
and come to their own satisfactory understanding of gender role.

By relegating psychosexual development to an ensemble role, we
do not mean to diminish its importance. We seek instead to contextualize it as one of many maturing systems that lead to a new
mental organization. As noted, all erogenous zones are potentially
active from infancy to adulthood, their coherence into an enduring constellation of love, sex, desire, and gender in the mind is *the*
oedipal achievement. But cognitive, semiotic, object relational,
self-regulatory, and affective developments are intrinsic to the
oedipal phase. Progression into new organization depends on the
interface of all these systems. The child's interest in the genital is
powerfully advanced by the recognition that it is this body part,
not hair length or clothing, that categorizes everyone as boy or girl,
man or woman (DeMarneffe, 1997). Thus in addition to its provision of pleasurable sensation, the genital's significance is radically
augmented by a cognitive advance. Children are certainly aware of
their sex and have already accrued and integrated ideas about its
meaning from familial and cultural sources, but the heightened sensation of the genital and how it pertains to "boyness" and "girlness"
is a new factor that becomes part of the assembly of sex and gender
elements.

Variations in the Oedipal Experience

Freud's original delineation of two oedipal complexes—the negative and positive—has been augmented by the recognition that differences in family configuration produce significant differences in the unconscious constellation. Even predating the contemporary transformation of parenting paradigms and reproductive methodology, the oedipal configuration was inevitably complicated by the variability of family structures. Siblings, divorce, parental death, and intra- or extra-familial adoption all become features that must be integrated into the triangulation of love relations, in addition to their other effects.

Siblings have been remarkably underrepresented in the developmental literature, with only a handful of papers examining their importance before the last decade. Exceptions are Graham's description of their role as "developmental companion(s)...(and) transferential shaper(s)" (Graham, 1988) and Neubauer's exploration of their influences on character organization (Neubauer, 1983). Graham's idea that the oedipal child's world is transformed "from a single planetary one that has the primary parental objects at the center and the sibling objects in orbit around them to that of a miniature universe of great complexity" (1988, p. 91) underscores sibling participation in the proliferation of oedipal configurations. Sharpe and Rosenblatt (1994) suggest that the historical tendency to consider siblings' roles as mere displacements from the parents obscures their primary position in oedipal triangles. Triangulation with a sibling as the object of desire or the rival takes on a new level of intensity, because siblings are peers who are unprotected by the "sacred" status of the parent (Loewald, 1979), both in regard to the incest taboo and the unleashing of aggression. Without the deep countervailing need to sanctify and preserve the relationship, triangles including siblings in the position of desired object or rival are fraught with the real potential for sex and aggression. There is less ambivalence and less tolerance for delayed gratification when the rival is a sibling, an equal, who is enjoying greater intimacy with the coveted parent right now. There is less terror about incest because, in desiring a sibling, the generational boundary is preserved. Moreover, the oedipal conflict with parents ultimately aids in the child's individuation and acceptance of such generational boundaries, but rivalry with a sibling does neither (Vivona, 2007). How can one differentiate from another who is so minimally different from the self? Indeed, Mitchell (2003) has proposed that a universal *sibling trauma* precedes the oedipal phase, when the child realizes that its position as beloved baby is not secure and is (typically) directly confronted with the mother's intimate exchange with the new baby. This foreshadowing of the primal scene is all the more galling because it involves a pleasure just recently in the child's possession—the mother's breast and the maternal embrace.

Contemporary Clarifications

There are many reasons that oedipal terminology has been so enduring. Outstanding among them is the fact that the oedipal phase comprises such a profound and transformative period of childhood, in which physical, semiotic, and emotional development explodes and passions flourish. The phase brings the child from unruly toddlerhood to the self-regulated, educable mental organization of latency, and ushers in the last significant addition to mental structure, that is, the superego. Although contemporary thinkers do not agree with the idea that psychosexuality is the major driver of development, most psychoanalytic schools concur that the oedipal phase and complex figure among Freud's enduring insights. His recognition of the remarkable shift in mental organization and the lasting impact of oedipal resolution on personality is central to a range of psychoanalytic theorizing. The importance of the oedipal phase and the complex that defines it continues as a unifying thread in psychoanalytic theories.

Theorists interested in the transforming culture around parenting differ, but most, implicitly or explicitly, endorse psychosexual development as an evolving system in childhood (Michels, 1999) and see that children's sexual researches, bodily interests, cognitive and emotional development, and emerging capacities bring them to a triangulated mental configuration of object relations that includes (and excludes) a "third." This momentous achievement expands the dyad and geometrically multiplies the mental challenges in the arenas of love relationships, rivalry, ambivalence, self-regulation, and the experience of guilt.

Implications for Mental Health and Psychopathology

Many theorists categorize psychopathology by positioning disorders along a preoedipal-oedipal continuum, based on the idea that the developmental accomplishments of the oedipal phase bring the personality into a higher-order neurotic level organization: Capacity for triadic whole-object relations, affective complexity and self-regulation, functional superego and guilt, mature ego defenses based on repression, and so on (Kernberg, 2005; Loewald, 1985). In this formulation, successful passage through the oedipal phase insures these developmental accomplishments, whereas their absence points to some earlier developmental phase wherein psychopathology began. According to some thinkers, "pre-oedipal" symptoms or personality organizations are primitive and disturbed, like psychoses and severe personality disorders (narcissistic or borderline), whereas oedipal level disorders are far more evolved and mature, with neurotic psychopathology.

Despite critiques emanating from a range of thinkers, this short-hand continues to appear in the literature. Taken literally, it assumes:

> ...that (1) a continuum of development is isomorphic with a continuum of pathology, (2) the origin of severe character pathology lies in the first three years of life, (3) there is a discontinuity between the pre-oedipal and oedipal years, such that certain fundamental phenomena (such as splitting, poorly integrated self-structure and narcissism) are transcended by the oedipal period, (4) 'object relations' refers to a unitary phenomenon or developmental line, (5) developmental sequences

in object relations are culturally invariant, and (6) clinical data from pathological adults are necessary and largely sufficient for constructing and evaluating theories of object-relational pathology and development. (Westen, 1990, p. 862)

Personality development begins in infancy and undergoes transformational steps. Adult psychopathology cannot be understood as the simple perpetuation of or regression to earlier forms, nor can the characterization of types of psychopathology be used to determine where in development they originate (Willick, 1983). Both health and psychopathology must be placed in the context of the totality of individual development and life experience, the overall ego organization, and the level of current functioning. They cannot be represented as proof of disruption or continuity of specific development moments. The idea of *regression*, conceptually linked to the continuum idea, is one that is commonly invoked but similarly inaccurate if taken literally (Dowling, 2004; Fosshage, 2010; Inderbitzin & Levy, 2000). When adult psychopathology is described as regressed, primitive, or a specific regression from oedipal conflict, implying a *fixation* at an earlier point in psychosexual development, such formulations require a second look. Adult psychopathology may resemble, but is not a regression to (that is, a return to), childhood mental organizations and naïve cognitions. Adult mental organization is not a layer, under which can be found previous ones: "The present is always emerging, always new, yet also always the outcome of the past" (Dowling, 2004, p. 193). Children do progress in roughly comparable sequences of states (Gilmore, 2008) or series of hierarchical mental organizations (Abrams, 1978), but those earlier mental organizations are not buried under the current one, available to be rediscovered at a later time or in moments of breakdown. Mental life exists as a "continuously constructed present" in which previous forms continue, contribute to the present moment, and, in a form inevitably shaped by development and current dynamics, can be reinterpreted and reutilized as part of the present repertoire (Dowling, 2004, pp. 201–202). Childhood mental states are never fully recreated in adult psychopathology, even while derivatives of childhood naïve cognitions and unconscious fantasy can be recognized in the adult. So even if the terminology of preoedipal and oedipal persists, it should not be interpreted concretely as an assertion of exactly when development went awry.

Another problem with the continuum theory as applied to oedipal level personality organization is that it gives a false picture of the child emerging from the oedipal phase. The notion of oedipal level personality organization, as it is typically used in evaluating personality disorders, does not really exist in terms of the regular transformations of childhood mental capacities. It implies a level of integration and maturity that is not achieved for many years following the waning of the Oedipus. For example, children well into latency continue to demonstrate "splitting" in their thinking about relationships and their feelings about others (Westen, 1989). The significance of the oedipal moment is that children's advancing developmental capacities allow them to appreciate a new level of environmental complexity—in terms of the dynamics of relationships—including the intense passions, rivalries, unrequited desires, and ambivalences swirling around and within them. The very advances that open their eyes to these intricacies—including symbolic thinking, mentalization, and self-regulation—come to their aid in managing them. But movement through this phase into latency does not imply the finalization of mental structure or the full maturation of any of these capacities. Although a new mental organization certainly appears in the postoedipal child, development is not complete and requires subsequent evolution to achieve its mature form (Novick & Novick, 1994). Moreover, it can be derailed by subsequent disruptions, arising from within (such as genetic predispositions and limitations) and from the environment.

The Impact of Pluralism on the Hegemony of the Oedipal Complex

Modern psychoanalytic theory is, of course, not singular, and today's many theoretical schools weigh the oedipal complex differently.

It remains of great importance in Kleinian and ego psychological thinking, in which it is consistently seen as a prime organizer of mental life, regardless of theoretical differences in developmental chronology (Gilmore, 2012). However, many schools of thought of more recent vintage have demoted oedipal conflict, albeit in different ways. Self-psychology, emerging in the 1970s (see Kohut, 1982) sees the traditional portrayal of intense intergenerational conflict as a manifestation of prior disturbance in the development of the self, whereas the relational schools, rising in the 1980s, shift the focus from psychosexual development and conflict toward a two-person psychology that privileges the role of relationships over drive and reality over intrapsychic unconscious fantasy (Seligman, 2003). Many of these schools—the self-psychological, the relational, the intersubjective are influenced by the rise of attachment theory. In some, this has resulted in the prioritization of infancy and mother–infant attunement. The oedipal complex as the centerpiece of human development has been criticized as either pathological or prescriptive and normative, in contrast to more open-ended notions of sexuality and gender development (Chodorow, 1994). Moreover, some contemporary thinkers suggest that the oedipal complex is simply no longer relevant on the basis of its grounding in conventional family structure and modes of conception, which are gradually being replaced by technology and changed sensibilities (Seligman, 1996).

Although the impact of such theoretical and societal changes is yet to be determined, a modified and expanded oedipal concept continues to provide an invaluable tool for understanding human development and the human mind. In the words of one highly regarded relationalist who continues to work with oedipal themes, "I am struck with the richness of the oedipal concept, how much ground [it] covers" (Altman, 1997, p. 739). Although not obscuring the multiple strands of development that converge in this period and the bidirectional nature of human interaction, the oedipal drama and its resolution, with their infinite variations, can be appreciated as a powerful attractor state achieved by developmental advances of this period, laying the groundwork for future personality organization.

We recognize the importance of the child's real circumstances and the role of significant others in shaping this drama, as well as ongoing developmental concerns, such as attachment, that can be drawn into the fray. As we demonstrate in the remaining chapters of this book, development certainly continues following this phase, and hugely important ego capacities, physical changes, psychological transformations, and experiences continue to reconfigure mental life. But the oedipal constellation, as a product of children's naïve cognition intersecting with veridical perceptions, wishful thinking, and the emergence of powerful impulses and feelings, becomes a rich source of unconscious fantasies, both universal and idiosyncratic (Erreich, 2003), that continue to influence the mind as development proceeds.

Summary

The oedipal phase, between three and six years, is a period of profound psychological development that generates a vast expansion of the child's potential for creative fantasy, emotional expression, self-regulation, and relationships. An intense emotional drama, the oedipal complex, unfolds within the child's family constellation, leaving an enduring impact on psychic life. Although contemporary thinkers have revised many aspects of Freud's original conceptualization, such as his views on female maturation, the oedipal phase is considered by many to be a centerpiece of psychoanalytic theorizing and a lens through which adult fantasy, relationships, and neuroses are understood.

A proliferation of symbolic functions, including the advent of narrative capacities, imagination and pretend play, and the acquisition of a theory of mind, support the emergence of complex fantasy, triadic relationships, and expanded resources for emotional self-regulation. Sexual and gender identity become defining features of the self; castration fears and fantasies gain intensity. Resolution of the oedipal drama yields a more abstract level of identification with the parents; internalization of parental standards and the

appearance of moral anxiety are foundational for a new mental agency, the superego, which facilitates the transition to latency.
   Key points about oedipal development include the following:

- The *oedipal phase* and the *oedipal complex* are linked but separate concepts. The former refers to a developmental period, typically between ages three and six. The complex represents an emotional drama, vis-à-vis central adult figures, which generates intense feelings of desire and jealousy. This early childhood experience persists as an enduring intrapsychic constellation.
- The development of symbolic capacities such as narrative language, complex imaginative play, and mentalization contributes to the transformation of the child's relationships, to self-regulatory resources and superego functions, and to a vastly expanded potential for mental fantasy.
- Sex and gender emerge as potent identifiers; bodily differences arouse intense interest as well as anxieties. The oedipal child manifests avid curiosity about parental sexual activity and reproductive functions; naïve observations and distortions are woven into enduring unconscious fantasies

References

Abrams, S. (1978). The teaching and learning of psychoanalytic developmental psychology. *Journal of the American Psychoanalytic Association, 26,* 87–406.

Altman, N. (1997). The case of Ronald: oedipal issues in the treatment of a seven-year-old boy. *Psychoanalytic Dialogues, 7,* 725–739.

Bernstein, D. (1990). Female genital anxieties, conflicts and typical mastery modes. *International Journal Psycho-Analysis, 71,* 151–165.

Bettelheim, B. (1975). Oedipal conflicts and resolutions: the knight in shining armor and the damsel in distress. In *The Uses of Enchantment: the Meaning and Importance of Fairy Tales* (pp. 111–116). New York: Random House.

Blum, H. P. (2010). Object relations in contemporary psychoanalysis: contrasting views. *Contemporary Psychoanalysis, 46*, 32–47.

Bretherton, I. (1990). Communication patterns, internal working models, and the intergenerational transmission of attachment relationships. *Infant Mental Health Journal, 11*, 237–252.

Carlson, S. M., Mandell, D. J., & Williams, L. (2004). Executive function and theory of mind: stability and prediction from ages two to three. *Developmental Psychology, 40*, 1105–1122.

Chodorow, N. (1994). *Femininities, Masculinities, Sexualities: Freud and Beyond.* Lexington, KY: University Press of Kentucky.

Cohen, D. J., Marans, S., Dahl, K., Marans, W., & Lewis, M. (1987). Analytic discussions with oedipal children. *Psychoanalytic Study of the Child, 42*, 59–83.

Cole, P., Armstrong, L. M., & Pemberton, C. K. (2010). The role of language in the development of emotional regulation. In S. Calkins & M. Bell (Eds.), *Child Development at the Intersection of Emotion and Cognition. Human Brain Development* (pp. 59–77). Washington, DC: American Psychological Association.

Corbett, K. (2001). Nontraditional family romance. *Psychoanalytic Quarterly, 70*, 599–624.

Denhan, S., Blair, K., De Mulder, E., Levitas, J., Sawyer, K. S., Auerbach-Major, S. T., et al. (2003). Preschoolers' emotional competence: pathway to social competence? *Child Development, 74*, 238–256.

DeMarneffe, D. (1997). Bodies and words: a study of young children's genital and gender knowledge. *Gender & Psychoanalysis, 2*, 3–33.

Dowling, A. S. (2004). A reconsideration of the concept of regression. *Psychoanalytic Study of the Child, 59*, 191–210.

Edgcumbe, R. & Burgner, M. (1975). The phallic-narcissistic phase—a differentiation between oedipal and preoedipal phases of development. *Psychoanalytic Study of the Child, 30*, 161–168.

Emde, R., Kubicek, L., & Oppenheim, D. (1997). Imaginative reality observed during early language development. *International Journal of Psychoanalysis, 78*, 115–133.

Erreich, A. (2003). A modest proposal: (re)defining unconscious fantasy. *Psychoanalytic Quarterly, 72*, 541–574.

Fein, G. G. (1981). Pretend play in childhood: an integrated review. *Child Development, 52*, 1095–1118.

Flavell, J. H., Flavell E. R., & Green, F. L. (1983). Development of the appearance-reality distinction. *Cognitive Psychology, 15*, 95–120.

Fonagy, P. & Target, M. (1996). Playing with reality: I. Theory of mind and the normal development of psychic reality. *International Journal of Psychoanalysis, 77,* 217–233.

Fosshage, J. L. (2010). Implicit and explicit dimensions of oedipal phenomenology: a reassessment. *Psychoanalytic Inquiry, 30,* 520–534.

Freud, S. (1905). Three essays on the theory of sexuality. In J. Strachey (Ed. and Trans.), *The Standard Edition of the Complete Psychological Works of Sigmund Freud* (Vol. 7, pp. 123–246). London: Hogarth Press.

Freud, S. (1920). Beyond the pleasure principle. In J. Strachey (Ed. and Trans.), *The Standard Edition of the Complete Psychological Works of Sigmund Freud,* (Vol. 18, pp. 1–64). London: Hogarth Press.

Freud, S. (1923). The infantile genital organization (an interpolation into the theory of sexuality). In J. Strachey (Ed. and Trans.), *The Standard Edition of the Complete Psychological Works of Sigmund Freud* (Vol. 19, pp. 139–146). London: Hogarth Press.

Gergely, G. (2000). Reapproaching Mahler: new perspectives on normal autism. *Journal of the American Psychoanalytic Association, 48,* 1197–1228.

Gilmore, K. (1998). Cloacal anxiety in female development. *Journal of American Psychoanalytic Association, 46,* 443–470.

Gilmore, K. (2005). Play in the psychoanalytic setting: ego capacity, ego state and vehicle for intersubjective exchange. *Psychoanalytic Study of the Child, 60,* 213–238.

Gilmore, K. (2008). Psychoanalytic developmental theory: a contemporary reconsideration. *Journal of American Psychoanalytic Association, 56,* 885–907.

Gilmore, K. (2011). Pretend play and development in early childhood (with implications for the oedipal phase). *Journal of American Psychoanalytic Association, 59,* 1157–1181.

Gilmore, K. (2012). Childhood experiences and the adult world. In G. O. Gabbard, B. E. Litowitz, & P. Williams (Eds.), *Textbook of Psychoanalysis* (2nd ed., pp. 117–131). Arlington, VA: American Psychiatric Publishing.

Ginot, E. (2012). Self-narratives and dysregulated affective states: the neuropsychological links between self-narratives, attachment, affect and cognition. *Psychoanalytic Psychology, 29,* 59–80.

Graham, I. (1988). The sibling object and its transferences: alternate organizer of the middle field. *Psychoanalytic Inquiry, 8,* 88–107.

Haden, C., Haine, R., & Fivush, R. (1997). Developing narrative structure in parent-child reminiscing across the preschool years. *Developmental Psychology, 33*, 295–307.

Harris, P. L., de Rosnay, M., & Pons, R. (2005). Language and children's understanding of mental states. *Current Directions in Psychological Science, 14*, 69–73.

Heineman, T. V. (2004). A boy and two mothers: new variations on an old theme or a new story of triangulation? Beginning thoughts on the psychosexual development of children in nontraditional families. *Psychoanalytic Psychology, 21*, 99–115.

Howe, N., Petraakos, H., Rinaldi, C., & LeFebvre, R. (2005). "This is a dog, you know...". Constructing shared meanings during sibling pretend play. *Child Development, 76*, 783–794.

Inderbitzin, L. B. & Levy, S. T. (2000). Regression and psychoanalytic technique: the concretization of a concept. *Psychoanalytic Quarterly, 69*, 195–223.

Jacobson, E. (1976). Female superego formation and the female castration conflict. *Psychoanalytic Quarterly, 45*, 525–538.

Jurist, E. L. (2005). Mentalized affectivity. *Psychoanalytic Psychology, 22*, 426–444.

Kernberg, O. (2005). Unconscious conflict in the light of contemporary psychoanalytic findings. *Psychoanalytic Quarterly, 74*, 65–68.

Knight, R. (2003). Margo and me II: The role of narrative building in child analytic technique. *Psychoanalytic Study of the Child, 58*, 133–164.

Kochanska, G., Coy, K. C., & Murray, K. T. (2001). The development of self-regulation in the first 4 years of life. *Child Development, 72*, 1091–1111.

Kohut, H. (1982). Introspection, empathy and the semi-circle of mental health. *International Journal of Psycho-analysis, 63*, 395–407.

Laible, D. & Song, J. (2006). Constructing emotional and relational understanding: the role of affect and mother-child discourse. *Merrill-Palmer Quarterly, 52*, 44–69.

Laible, D. & Thompson, R. A. (2000). Mother-child discourse, attachment security, shared positive affect and early conscience development. *Child Development, 71*, 1424–1440.

Lillard, A. S., Lerner, M. D., Hopkins, E. J., Dore, R. A., Smith, E. D., & Palmquist, C. M. (2013). The impact of pretend play on children's development: a review of the evidence. *Psychological Bulletin, 139*, 1–34.

Loewald, H. (1985). Oedipus complex and development of self. *Psychoanalytic Quarterly, 54,* 435–443.

Loewald, H. W. (1970). Psychoanalytic theory and psychoanalytic process. *Psychoanalytic Study Child, 25,* 45–68.

Loewald, H. W. (1979). The waning of the Oedipus complex. *Journal of the American Psychoanalytic Association, 27,* 751–775.

Lyons-Ruth, K. (2006). Play, precariousness and the negotiation of shared meaning: a developmental perspective on child psychotherapy. *Journal of Infant, Child and Adolescent Psychotherapy, 5,* 142–145.

Mahler, M. (1971). A study of the separation-individuation process and its application to borderline phenomena in the psychoanalytic situation. *Psychoanalytic Study of the Child, 26,* 403–424.

Mahler, M., Pine, F., & Bergman, A. (1975). *The Psychological Birth of the Human Infant: Symbiosis & Individuation.* New York: Basic Books.

Main, M. (2000). The organized categories of infant, child and adult attachment: flexible vs inflexible attention under attachment-related stress. *Journal of American Psychoanalytic Association, 48,* 1055–1096.

Marans, S., Mayes, L., Cicchetti, D., Dahl, K., Marans, W., & Cohen, D. J. (1991). The child-psychoanalytic play interview: a technique for studying thematic content. *Journal of American Psychoanalytic Association, 39,* 1015–1036.

Mayer, E. L. (1985). "Everybody must be just like me": observations on female castration anxiety. *International Journal of Psycho-Analysis, 66,* 331–347.

Mayes, L. C. & Cohen, D. J. (1992). The development of a capacity for imagination in early childhood. *Psychoanalytic Study of the Child, 47,* 23–47.

Mayes, L. C. & Cohen, D. J. (1996). Children's development of theory of mind. *Journal American Psychoanalytic Association, 44,* 117–142.

Meyer, J. & Tuber, S. (1989). Intrapsychic and behavioral correlates of the phenomenon of imaginary companions in young children. *Psychoanalytic Psychology, 6,* 151–168.

Michels, R. (1999) Psychoanalysts' theories. In P. Fonagy, A. Cooper, & R. Wallerstein (Eds.), *Psychoanalysis on the Move: The Work of Joseph Sandler.* New Library of Psychoanalysis (Vol 35, pp. 187–200). London: Hogarth Press.

Migden, S. (1998). Dyslexia and self-control: an ego psychoanalytic perspective. *Psychoanalytic Study of the Child, 53,* 282–299.

Moll, H. & Tomasello, M. (2012). Three year olds understand appearance and reality—just not about the same object at the same time. *Developmental Psychology, 48,* 1124–1132

Moll, H., Metzoff, A. N., Merzsch, K., & Tomasello, M. (2013). Taking versus confronting visual perspectives in preschool children. *Developmental Psychology, 49,* 646–654.

Mitchell, J. (2003). *Siblings: Sex and Violence.* Cambridge, UK: Polity Press.

Nelson, K. (1996). *Language in Cognitive Development. The Emergence of the Mediated Mind.* Cambridge, MA: Cambridge University Press.

Neubauer, P. B. (1983). The importance of the sibling experience. *Psychoanalytic Study of the Child, 38,* 325–336.

Neubauer, P. B. (1987). The many meanings of play: Introduction. *Psychoanalytic Study of the Child, 42,* 3–11.

Novick, K. K. & Novick, J. (1994). Postoediapl transformations: laterncy, adolescence, and pathogenesis. *Journal of the American Psychoanalytic Association, 42,* 143–169.

Olesker, W. (1998). Female genital anxieties: views from the nursery and the couch. *Psychoanalytic Quarterly, 67,* 276–294.

Oppenheim, D., Koren-Karie, N., & Sagi-Schwartz, A. (2007). Emotional dialogues between mother and child at 4.5 and 7.5 years: relations with children's attachment at 1 year. *Child Development, 78,* 38–52.

Parens, H. (1990). On the girl's psychosexual development: reconsiderations suggested from direct observation. *Journal of the American Psychoanalytic Association, 38,* 743–772.

Peterson, I. T., Bates, J. E., D'Onofrio, B. M., Coyne, C. A., Lansford, J. E., Dodge, R. A., et al. (2013). Language ability predicts the development of behavior problems in children. *Journal of Abnormal Psychology, 122,* 542–557.

Piaget, J. (1926). *The Language and Thought of the Child.* London: Kegan Paul, Trench, Trubner & Co.

Ruffman, T., Slade, L., & Crowe, E. (2002). The relationship between children's and mother's mental state language and theory of mind understanding. *Child Development, 73,* 734–751.

Seligman, D. (1996). Commentaries. *Journal of the American Psychoanalytic Association, 44,* 430–446.

Seligman, S. (2003). The developmental perspective in relationship psychoanalysis. *Contemporary Psychoanalysis, 39,* 477–508.

Sharpe, S. & Rosenblatt, A. (1994). Oedipal sibling triangles. *Journal of the American Psychoanalytic Association, 42,* 491–523.

Simon, B. (1991). Is the oedipus complex still the cornerstone of psychoanalysis? Three obstacles to answering the question. *Journal of the American Psychoanalytic Association, 39,* 641–668.

Singer, D. G. & Singer, J. L. (1992). *The House of Make Believe.* Cambridge, MA: Harvard University Press.

Vivona, J. M. (2007). Sibling differentiation, identity development, and the lateral dimension of psychic life. *Journal of the American Psychoanalytic Association, 60,* 55, 1191–1215.

Vygotsky, L. S. (1978). *Mind in Society: The Development of Higher Psychological Processes.* Cambridge, MA: Harvard University Press.

Wellman, H. M., Phillips, A. T., & Rodriguez, T. (2000). Young children's understanding of perception, desire and emotion. *Child Development, 71,* 895–912.

Westen, D. (1989). Are "primitive" object relations really preoedipal? *American Journal Orthopsychiatry, 59,* 331–345.

Westen, D. (1990). Towards a revised theory of borderline object relations: contributions of empirical research. *International Journal of Psycho-Analysis, 71,* 661–693.

Weinberg, E. (2006). Mentalization, affect regulation and development of the self. *Journal of the American Psychoanalytic Association, 54,* 251–269.

Willick, M. S. (1983). On the concept of primitive defenses. *Journal of the American Psychoanalytic Association, 31S,* 175–200.

Wimmer, H. & Perner, J. (1983). Beliefs about beliefs: representations and constraining functions of wrong beliefs in children's understanding of deception. *Cognition, 13,* 105–128.

Winsler, A. (2003). Vygotskian perspectives in early childhood education: introduction to special issue. *Early Education & Development, 14,* 253–270.

Woolley, J. & Wellman, H. (1993). Origin and truth: young children's understanding of imaginative mental representations. *Child Development, 64,* 1–17.

5

Latency: The Era of Learning, Autonomy, and Peer Relationships

Overview

The latency phase spans the ages between six and ten, roughly corresponding to the years of grade school; indeed, the highly visible markers of latency are the school child's absorption in learning and passion for achievement. This period of development, during which the child is uniquely available to the transmission of culturally valued norms and skills, is universally acknowledged as the "age of reason" or the "era of industry" (Erikson, 1950; Mahon, 1991; Shapiro, 1976). Increasingly stable superego capacities, along with an underlying cognitive revolution, create a vastly enhanced potential for separation and autonomous functioning. The child's propensity for reality-based situations, such as learning and peer socialization, is a fundamental distinction between latency and the previous oedipal phase. In contrast to the subsequent stages of adolescent development, bodily maturation proceeds at a slow and consistent pace, exerting minimal pressure on the child's mental life.

The mind of the latency child is characterized by an unprecedented capacity for logical reasoning, a consolidation of parental identifications, and a proliferation of defensive resources such as repression, sublimation, intellectualization, and fantasy formation. Together, these advances in ego and superego functioning reinforce reality testing and self–other differentiation, facilitate relations beyond the family, and help transform infantile wishes and impulses into latency-phase pursuits and daydreams (Novick & Novick, 1994, 2004; Piaget & Inhelder, 1969; Sarnoff, 1971). Prolonged periods of separation from parents and immersion in peer socialization further serve to reinforce oedipal prohibitions and self-control. Amplified societal demands—expectations for learning, compliance, prosocial behavior—interface with the child's newfound abilities and mounting desire for independence and friendship, creating a developmental period that is synonymous with cooperation, diligence, and productivity, and in which peer norms begin to exert a powerful influence.

Historic Views of Latency

Early conceptualizations of latency (Freud, 1905a, 1924) posit a relatively dormant period in the biphasic development of mature sexuality, functioning as a lull between the oedipal phase and adolescence; defining characteristics of this period include the ascendancy of secondary process thinking, the dominance of the reality principle, and the reduction of drive pressures. Dissolution of the oedipal complex, which succumbs to repression, ushers in the latency phase; identifications, primarily with same-sex parental authority figures, create the foundation for superego functioning and ensure the erection of moral barriers against oedipal wishes. The combined presence of infantile amnesia, superego, and ego ideal (heirs to the positive and negative oedipal complex) maintain the psychic structure of latency. In this view, latency represents a temporary "truce" between instincts and ego: the comparative quiescence of drives provides the child with a period in which to consolidate ego capacities before the re-awakening of sexuality in preadolescence (Sandler & Freud, 1984).

Subsequent revisions of latency, however, shift away from the concept of dormancy and postulate a phase of ongoing, foundational mental development. Moreover, notions of singular causality, in this case the dissolution of the oedipal complex by fear of castration, are mostly abandoned in favor of more complex etiologies. The child's prodigious cognitive advances and the proliferation of symbolic capacities are seen as major contributors to a distinct latency psychic structure, maintained largely by fantasy formation, sublimation, and repression (Etchegoyen, 1993; Hartmann, Kris, & Loewenstein, 1949; Hartmann & Loewenstein, 1962; Sarnoff, 1971; Shapiro, 1976). Division of latency into early and later periods reflects recognition of a more gradual consolidation of the superego, beginning but certainly not complete at the close of the oedipal phase and requiring the child's continuing adjustment to internal moral conflicts. Masturbatory urges and fantasies are theorized to be only partially repressed in the initial phase of latency (Bornstein, 1951). Thus, early assumptions about the total destruction of the oedipal complex were adjusted such that suppression of sexual fantasies and impulses is viewed as relative rather than complete. The child's elaborate use of symbolization, including daydreams, jokes, and rhymes, provides multiple channels for the expression of ongoing oedipal fantasy in more or less disguised form (Mahon, 1991; Sarnoff, 1971).

Contemporary theorizing further broadens the array of interacting systems, examining the confluences of biology, family, and culture that contribute to the characteristic qualities of latency, as well as the synergistic relationship between the child's expanding ego capacities and environmental opportunities and expectations. Moreover, twenty-first century writers have new data that elucidate the operation of neurocognitive factors in such phenomena as infantile amnesia: Long viewed by classical psychoanalysts as a cornerstone of postoedipal functioning, the process of prelatency repression is now understood in the context of developing memory systems. Very early experiences are encoded by implicit (procedural), rather than explicit memory, making them inaccessible to recollection by a transformed mental organization (Brickman, 2008). The impact of environmental vicissitudes, such as prevailing cultural norms, the pressures of latency peer society, and patterns of gender segregation have also been integrated with existing theories of the latency phase (for examples, see Bernstein, 2001; Friedman, & Downey, 2000). Moreover, as psychoanalysis has increasingly interfaced with neurodevelopmental research, the powerful effects of learning differences and deficits emerge as enduring influences on the latency youngster's sense of self and capacity for self-regulation (Arkowitz, 2002; Gilmore, 2002; Weinstein & Saul, 2005).

In addition, the significantly earlier onset of puberty, access to new forms of socialization, information, and overstimulating content, both sexual and violent, through internet usage appears to be affecting the sanctity of the latency period as a time of instinctual quiescence. The impact of the internet on prepubertal children has yet to receive the research attention focused on adolescence, but it is increasingly recognized as a potent factor in latency development (Livingstone, 2003; McColgan & Giardino, 2005).

The Phases of Latency

The division of latency into early and late subphases, roughly capturing the years six through eight and then eight through ten, respectively, reflects highly visible distinctions in the child's capacity for autonomous functioning. Although individual progression through this period is extremely variable, subject not only to environmental provision, but also to the child's learning and self-regulatory endowment, we continue to find that such divisions are useful in identifying common transitions and evolution of developmental expectations. Certain theorists such as Knight (2005, 2011) posit three identifiable sub-phases for latency, marked by steps in the child's capacity for independence and self-regulation. However, in our opinion, the final subphase, spanning the years roughly between 10 and 12 has been so penetrated by increasingly early pubertal changes and the "tweening" effect of contemporary culture[1] that it merits the designation of preadolescence, described in chapter 6.

Within the psychoanalytic literature, these phase demarcations largely signify stages in the child's gradual consolidation of superego functioning and cognitive organization. During the initial postoedipal years, internalization of moral authority is shaky, leading to frequent disruptions in self-control and externalization of superego conflicts (Bornstein, 1951; Sarnoff, 1971). In the memorable words of one latency theorist, the young child experiences unfamiliar superego pressures as a "foreign body" in the psyche (Bornstein, 1951). The emergent cognitive style of this age group, which tends toward logical but categorical thinking, further contributes to moral rigidity and rule-bound attitudes (Piaget, 1932; Piaget & Inhelder, 1969). As the child progresses through latency, better self-regulation—supported by an underlying expansion of symbolic thinking—is indicated by decidedly more fluid and autonomous moral reasoning, greater stability of self-control and a pronounced turn toward socialization beyond the family.

Consistent with the notion of the superego as an "open system," the child's moral and self-regulatory style and functioning are subject to the shaping influence of the cultural surround (Novick & Novick, 2004). Both the school and home environments scaffold the second phase of latency by introducing more challenging standards and expectations. Within the American educational system, at around age eight, or during third grade, emphasis on rote skills transitions toward more abstract, complex tasks that require planning, organization, and collaboration. Such endeavors require a greater level of self-responsibility and collaboration in group projects. Simultaneously, the child often experiences a push from parents toward greater self-control and immersion in group activities and competitive pursuits.

Early latency is dominated by the child's precarious state of self-management, the novelty of guilty feelings, and the susceptibility to disruption of autonomous functioning. Environmental demands, especially those of school, are often experienced as overwhelming and unjust. A recently acquired sense of morality is governed by harsh, concrete, and unyielding self-chastisements, creating enormous conflict and giving rise to a palpable "emergency situation" (Bornstein, 1951). Relief is sought through the phase-appropriate defense of *externalization*, wherein inner prohibitions are relegated to outside sources of authority, such as teachers, from whom the child elicits punishment (Furman, 1980). Despite, or because of, the young child's highly inconsistent self-regulation, others' misdeeds are routinely called out: Behaviors such as tattling reach peak frequency (Loke, Heyman, & Gorgie, 2011).

During the immediate postoedipal phase, the child's fears of regression are unremitting and intense. Indeed, a sensitive form of defense analysis that specifically seeks to avoid unnecessary exposure of unconscious impulses is applied to this age-group (Bornstein, 1951; Hoffman, 2007). Rote, repetitive activities and obsessional phenomena are employed in an effort to ward off potential disruptions in self-control and to suppress prelatency impulses. Not only does the child's cognitive maturation makes possible the proliferation of such defenses, but activities involving relentless counting, classifying, collecting, and rule-bound games are highly valued and reinforced in the academic and social surround (Chused, 1999; Hartmann, Kris, & Loewenstein, 1949; Sarnoff, 1971). No child analyst has failed to encounter the latency youngster's affinity for structured activities and powerful avoidance of stimulating, open-ended fantasy, play, and dreams (Harley, 1962).

The later subphase of latency marks a transition toward a greater sense of separateness and more autonomous self-control (Knight, 2005, 2011). The eight- to ten-year-old is manifestly more competent, skilled, and self-possessed. Identifications with adults' standards and ideals are increasingly stable and self-generated, emotional self-regulation is more reliable and the child is less dependent on external provision of boundaries and punishments. At the same time, idealization of the parents begins to decline, and the child gains awareness that adults are fallible and their prohibitions are not law (Nobes & Pawson, 2003; Piaget, 1932). Foreshadowing the adolescent phase to come, the norms and self-made rules of the peer group begin to hold sway. The child's moral reasoning is less rigid and more abstract, characterized by such notions as reciprocity, cooperation, and individual responsibility. These various developments fuel and enable a fuller immersion in the social group and a facility for organized peer activities (e.g., hobbies, clubs, teams). Mentalization capacities are more automatic and fluid, allowing the child to grasp multiple perspectives and comprehend complex social situations (Jemerin, 2004). Moreover, the older child's vastly expanded symbolization, cognitive, and motor skills provide burgeoning opportunities for sublimation. Typical, latency-phase pursuits such as reading, research, creative writing, and sports function as socially sanctioned outlets for sublimated aggressive, competitive, or scoptophilic impulses.

Cognition and Learning in Latency

Cognitive Reorganization and Social Reasoning in Latency

The advent of logic and abstract mental reasoning, often referred to as entry into the period of *concrete operations*, is a universally demonstrated achievement of latency (Piaget & Inhelder, 1969; Suizzo, 2000). The hallmark of intellectual functioning during this phase is *decentering*, a capacity for objective reasoning in which thinking is detached from perceptual context. The increasing use of thought as trial action releases the child from egocentric, perceptually bound appraisals of both the physical and social world, constituting a powerful tool for self-regulation and behavioral inhibition. Underlying maturation of the prefrontal cortex, which functions to integrate personal goals with information about current context, facilitates the child's rapid acquisition of rules and structured activities (Bunge & Zelazo, 2006). A greater awareness of pragmatic facts and constraints, such as time, further contributes to a sense of reality and supports the child's new affinity for plans and projects.

The acquisition of organized, logical mental actions (or operations) is demonstrable in the latency child's growing ability to classify, add, and subtract without manipulation of objects. Such fundamental intellectual exercises are highly valued and promoted in the classroom and in turn fuel phase-typical pursuits like collecting and organizing. A grasp of abstract concepts, such as reversibility, enables the child to realize that essential characteristics (e.g., the mass of an object) are invariant despite superficial transformations. With diminished egocentrism, the latency child is increasingly able to consider multiple aspects of problems and contemplate diverse perspectives, without being unduly influenced by a single, salient factor. Historically, such advances in abstract thinking were assessed via the classic Piagetian tasks of conservation: For example, at around age seven, children verbally reason that a volume of liquid that has been poured from one container to a second of differing contour is not fundamentally altered (Piaget & Inhelder, 1969).

The process of decentering transforms relational capacities, expanding the child's theories of human behavior and enabling more complex interpretations of interpersonal events. In early latency, social thinking and moral judgments retain a rigid, conventional quality. Complex concepts, such as gender, tend to be viewed categorically; indeed, gender stereotyping reaches a peak in early latency, when the child's newly acquired capacity for classification initially fosters an either/or approach to personal characteristics (Martin & Ruble, 2004). Similarly, perceived rules and moral standards are governed by absolutism and are subject to simplistic interpretation; morality is closely aligned with adult authority and transgressions are measured by expected levels of punishment (Piaget, 1932).

As the child progresses through latency, however, a shift toward greater mental freedom and a sense of people's individuality emerges. Although basic theory of mind capacities (e.g., false belief tasks) are grasped at the age of four, as discussed in chapter 4, a more robust ability to decenter the self from infantile egocentricity is achieved only during middle childhood, leading to higher-order mental state knowledge than that associated with the preschool years. The older child achieves a greater facility to adopt others' perspectives and to keep in mind the multiple dimensions of complex social–emotional experience. Abstract concepts, such as invariance, inform social reasoning. The child realizes that inherent character traits, such as generosity, are enduring and can be used to make predictions about others' conduct (Alvarez, Ruble, & Bolger, 2001). Individuals are increasingly seen as unique and complex, and not merely as members of discrete categories such as male or female (Abrams, 2011). Moreover, although mentalization is inextricably linked to the early mother–child bond, the latency child's social–emotional understanding is an internalized, autonomous capacity that functions outside of the dyadic relationship (Jemerin, 2004). The older child is equipped to interpret the behavior of social groups and manage the inevitable conflicts and dilemmas that ensue among peers; simultaneously, the daily experience of latency, marked by collaboration in classroom groups, clubs, teams, and social communities conducted at a remove from parents, provides practice and reinforcement of developing skills.

School and Learning

The sweeping cognitive changes of latency create an unprecedented potential for systematic learning. Within the classroom environment, the child's newly emergent abilities to solve problems, internalize skills, and make plans are unceasingly practiced and assessed, making academic competence an increasingly prominent source of self-esteem. Within the empiric literature, the child's availability for learning is seen as resting upon the development of effortful control, a set of integrative, *executive functions* (see glossary) that guide goal-directed behavior and create freedom from internal disruption; these include managing and shifting attention, planning, voluntarily inhibiting responses, filtering distractions, and applying working memory capacities. The presence of cognitive controls is linked to successful negotiation of myriad latency tasks, such as adjustment to the structured demands of grade school, behavioral self-management, and positive peer relations (Eisenberg, Spinrad, & Eggum, 2010; Kochanska & Knaack, 2003; Luna et al., 2004; Ponitz et al., 2009). Although not inherent to the psychoanalytical lexicon, cognitive controls are currently recognized as a key component of ego development. Deficiencies in executive functioning, manifested by children with neurodevelopmental disorders such as attention deficit hyperactivity disorder (ADHD), are posited to create serious ego impairments, predisposing the child to dysregulation and social isolation (Cione et al., 2011; Gilmore, 2002).

As the child transitions from kindergarten to the more formal requirements of grade school academics, problems with learning and self-management become more visible. Common learning impediments, such as dyslexia, visual-motor delays, or attentional deficits are correlated with ongoing developmental and functional disturbances in such areas as self–object differentiation, behavioral self-control, self-regard, and academic progress (Barkley, 2006; Rothstein, 1998). Language-based delays, such as those hypothesized to interfere with reading, impede the child's access to higher-order, abstract processes, and limit the use of inner speech and verbal self-directives for behavioral self-control (Arkowitz, 2002; Frijling-Schreuder, 1972; Weinstein & Saul, 2005). Moreover, impediments to latency-phase pursuits such as reading, writing, and athletics, restrict channels for sublimation, eroding both emotional regulation and self-esteem. When these pursuits involve group socialization, the child's interpersonal development is also affected.

Symbolization and Fantasy in Latency Development

The latency child's avid pursuit of reality-based tasks and achievements is a quintessential feature of this phase, distinguishing it from the magical, imaginary mental world of the oedipal period. Playfulness and pretend outlets, such as theater, persist into latency and well beyond, but symbolic play recedes as the school-aged child turns toward structured projects, collections, hobbies, and rule-bound social games (Piaget, 1962; Solnit, 1998). Nonetheless, fantasy formation is a universal feature and a chief defense of the latency period (Sarnoff, 1971). Elaborate daydreams and absorption in popular, serialized stories provide outlets and transformations of prelatency wishes while also assuaging the novel discomfort of guilty feelings. In the latter phase of latency, as the child confronts frustrating tasks, disappointing outcomes, down-to-earth self-appraisals, and unfavorable comparisons with age-mates, imaginary contents are less fanciful and more realistic, reflecting the child's cognitive advances and desires for real-life adventures and achievements. Such fantasies, often grandiose in nature, help motivate the child to persist at rote, sometimes tedious exercises and mastery of skills (Novick & Novick, 1996). As latency draws to a close, the pleasurable benefits of fantasy decline. The young adolescent begins to seek direct satisfaction of impulses through action and ultimately via sexual contact (Battin & Mahon, 2009; Sarnoff, 1971).

The child's capacity for reading and comprehension of complex narratives widens exposure to a range of beloved latency stories. Traditionally, these feature plucky, clever children who outsmart and outperform adults. Inevitably, the protagonists are bereft of parental company: They are orphaned, abandoned, kidnapped, or just plain left alone (Weinstein & Shustorovich, 2011). Transparent story themes involve autonomy, peer friendship, separation, and magical transformations, all contents that directly relate to the child's sense of having been pushed from the family out into a harsh and unfair world (Knight, 2005). Some form of *family romance*, a fantasy of being the true offspring of other, more glamorous, noble, or important parents is consolidated in middle childhood and commonly represented in such narratives. This universal latency fantasy represents the child's mourning for the idealized parents of early childhood and assuages a growing disillusionment with the self and the adult world (A. Freud, 1963; Kaplan, 1974).

Other forms of symbolization, such as joking and rhymes, provide additional outlets for sexual and aggressive urges. Indeed, Freud (1905b) noted the suitability of the latency mind for joking, owing to the presence of recently repressed and only weakly inhibited instincts that continue to seek expression (Clowes, 1996). The older child's palpable pleasure in sexually themed jokes and rhymes, typically relished in group situations, reveals the ongoing pressure of oedipal wishes and impulses. These activities serve multiple purposes, providing discharge for prohibited urges while simultaneously reinforcing incest taboos and cementing group bonds (Clowes, 1996; Goldings, 1974).

Family and Peer Relationships

For the duration of latency, relations with parents remain close and cooperative, largely without the signs of friction that begin to surface during preadolescence. Parents retain moral authority and continue to exert a major influence on the child's overall functioning: A history of secure attachment, in combination with ongoing parental support and behavioral modeling, correlates with positive social adjustment and good self-regulatory capacities during the years of middle childhood (Contreras et al., 2000; Goodman, Bartlett, & Stroh, 2013; Main, Kaplan, & Cassidy, 1985). However, greater awareness of reality and exposure to individuals beyond the family accelerates the loss of parental idealization. The child begins to seek ancillary sources of identification and admiration via adults in positions of power, such as teachers and coaches. Increasingly, the peer group functions as a balance to adult figures of authority, providing the child with companionship as well as a contrasting set of rules and expectations.

Establishing peer bonds is a central developmental task of latency. Indeed, a number of theorists posit the grade school years as a critical period for peer connection: A state of "friendedness" at ages eight or nine tends to persist, whereas peer rejection during middle childhood is associated with ongoing social ostracism, loneliness, and difficulty with social–emotional adjustment in early adolescence (Pedersen et al., 2007). The latency child's autonomous self-regulation emerges as a decisive predictor of social success. Behavioral self-control is empirically linked to forming friendships, whereas disruptive behavior predisposes the child to peer rejection and correlates with low numbers of friends during grade school (Kochanska & Knaack, 2003; Pedersen et al., 2007).

In sharp distinction to the parent–child experience, peer-to-peer unions offer a unique opportunity for equality and shared interests in a relationship that lacks a fully mature and committed partner. The expectations of the cohort exert new pressures for perspective taking and behavioral conformity with peer norms (Bemporad, 1984; Friedman & Downey, 2008). Rule-bound group and dyadic games provide needed practice for socialization and collaboration (Piaget & Inhelder, 1969). In addition, socially acceptable venues like competitive sports serve as outlets for aggression and jealousy while maintaining separation of such impulses from their original parental objects. As peer relationships are consolidated, they serve as meaningful and compensatory substitutes as the postoedipal child suffers a gradual disillusionment with the parents and mourns the decline of infantile object ties (Bemporad, 1984; Knight, 2005, 2011; Loewald, 1979).

Latency society is largely composed of sex-segregated friendships and groups with distinctly asymmetric gender-based expectations and conventions. Such divisions are both biologically determined and socially constructed. Once generated, children themselves are active in promoting and reinforcing gender partitions and exclusionary rules (Friedman & Downey, 2008; Sroufe et al., 1993). Boys' groups are notoriously larger, action-oriented, hierarchically organized and rejecting toward both girls and adults; preferred activities reflect male fantasies of danger, exploration, adventure, and competition (Friedman & Downey, 2008; Maccoby, 2002). Girls' groups are characterized by more open and cooperative attitudes, but with a tendency toward exclusive cliques; typical female play tends to reflect such themes as romance and childrearing. Furthermore, girls are more likely to engage in the sharing of secrets and other private, intimate information, whereas boys tend to be less informed about their male friends' private lives (Kulish, 2002; Maccoby, 2002). Participation in sex-based groups is a key source of "gender-valued self-esteem" during late childhood (Friedman & Downey, 2008, p. 153). The authority of such groups to set standards and confer status gathers intensity as the child approaches the preadolescent phase of development.

Summary

The latency phase, spanning the ages between six and ten, is synonymous with the "age of reason" or the "era of industry"; once viewed as a time of relative psychic dormancy, this period of childhood is now seen as characterized by sweeping changes in cognition, self-regulation, and socialization. The gradual internalization of superego prohibitions and a vastly expanded repertoire of ego capacities and defenses—including sublimation and fantasy formation—facilitate a phase of unprecedented autonomy and learning, wherein an extravagant array of culturally valued skills and standards is rapidly acquired.

The division of latency into early (six to eight years) and late (eight to ten) phases marks a shift in cognitive reorganization and superego consolidation: after an initially shaky postoedipal period, noteworthy for frequent lapses in self-control, the child manifests an increasingly stable and autonomous inner moral voice. Failures in the development of emotional self-regulation emerge as key risk factors in latency. Such ego impairments, which are linked to insecure parent–child bonds, environmental overstimulation, as well as neurodevelopmental disorders, threaten to disrupt foundational social and academic experiences. As the parents are de-idealized and the bonds of friendship assume greater importance, a decisive turn away from the family and toward group socialization foreshadows the rise of the peer group in preadolescence.

For those working clinically with latency-aged children, the following points are especially relevant:

- During the early phase of latency (six to eight years), children's capacity for emotional and behavioral self-management is brittle. Newly emergent neurodevelopmental abilities (e.g., planning, organization, logical problem-solving) facilitate self-regulation, but early superego functions are unreliable and cause the child to often feel on the brink of a loss of self-control.
- Externalization, wherein the child relies on environmental responses during times of inner discomfort, is a normative defense of this age group.

- Interpretative work with young latency children is geared to avoid exposure of deep fantasies and fears.
- The later phase of latency (eight to ten years) is marked by more stable self-control and a decisive turn toward the peer group. Compensatory fantasies, such as versions of the family romance, help assuage the growing awareness of reality and of personal and parental limitations.
- An underlying cognitive transformation, beginning at around age seven, contributes to the latency child's affinity for learning, rule-bound games, and multiple skills. The child's intellectual shifts create diverse defensive potentials, including a variety of sublimations.
- In the clinical setting, the latency child may avoid the regressive pull of fantasy play and veer toward more rote, rule-based activities.
- Learning challenges may significantly impact the school-aged child's sense of self and limit access to age-appropriate subliminatory channels, affecting developing capacities for emotional self-regulation.

Notes

1. Although the term was used to designate what amounts to emerging adulthood (20–33) by J. R. R. Tolkien, it has been a customary term for children between 10 and 12, who are considered an important demographic for advertisers (see Aucoin, 2005).

References

Abrams, D. (2011). Wherein lies children's intergroup bias? Egocentrism, social understanding and social projection. *Child Development, 82,* 1579–1593.

Alvarez, J. M., Ruble, D. N., & Bolger, N. (2001). Trait understanding or evaluatative reasoning? An analysis of children's behavioral predictions. *Child Development, 72,* 1409–1425.

Arkowitz, S. W. (2002). On the over-stimulated state of dyslexia: perception, knowledge and learning. *Journal of the American Psychoanalytic Association, 48*, 1491–1520.

Aucoin, D. (2005). Too old for toys, too young for boys. *Boston Globe*, Feb 2. Accessed September 2013: http://www.boston.com/news/globe/living/articles/2005/02/02/too_old_for_toys_too_young_for_boys/

Barkley, R. A. (2006). *Attention-Deficit/Hyperactivity Disorder: A Handbook for Diagnosis and Treatment* (3rd ed.). New York: Guilford.

Battin, D. & Mahon, E. (2009). Seeing the light. *Psychoanalytic Quarterly, 78*, 107–122.

Bemporad, J. R. (1984). From attachment to affiliation. *American Journal of Psychoanalysis, 44*, 79–92.

Bernstein, A. (2001). A note on the passing of the latency period. *Modern Psychoanalysis, 26*, 283–287.

Bornstein, B. (1951). On latency. *Psychoanalytic Study of the Child, 6*, 279–285.

Brickman, H. R. (2008). Living within the cellular envelope: subjectivity and self from an evolutionary neuro-psychoanalytic perspective. *Journal of the American Academy of Psychoanalysis, 36*, 317–341.

Bunge, S. A. & Zelazo, P. D. (2006). A brain-based account of the development of rule use in childhood. *Current Directions in Psychological Science, 15*, 118–121.

Chused, J. F. (1999). Obsessional manifestations in childhood. *Psychoanalytic Study of the Child, 54*, 219–232.

Cione, G. F., Coleburn, J. D., Fertuck, E. A., & Fraenkel, P. (2011). Psychodynamic play therapy with a six-year-old African-American boy with ADHD. *Journal of Infant, Child and Adolescent Psychotherapy, 10*, 130–143.

Clowes, E. K. (1996). Oedipal themes in latency: analysis of the farmer's daughter joke. *Psychoanalytic Study of the Child, 51*, 436–454.

Contraras, J. M., Kerns, K. A., Weimer, B. L., Gentzler, A. L., & Tomich, P. L. (2000). Emotion regulation as a mediator of association between mother-child attachment and peer relations in middle childhood. *Journal of Family Psychology, 14*, 111–124.

Eisenberg, N., Spinarad, T. L., & Eggum, N. D. (2010). Emotion-related self-regulation and its relation to children's maladjustments. *Annual Review of Clinical Psychology, 6*, 495–525.

Erikson, E. H. (1950). *Childhood and Society* (2nd ed.). New York: Norton.

Etchegoyen, A. (1993). Latency—a reappraisal. *International Journal of Psychoanalysis, 74*, 347–357.

Frijling-Schreuder, E. C. (1972). The vicissitudes of aggression in normal development, in childhood neurosis and in childhood psychosis. *International Journal of Psychoanalysis, 53*, 185–190.

Friedman, R. C. & Downey, J. I. (2000). The psychobiology of late childhood. *Journal of the American Academy of Psychoanalysis, 28*, 431–448.

Friedman, R. C. & Downey, J. I. (2008). Sexual differentiation of behavior. *Journal of the American Psychoanalytic Association, 56*, 147–175.

Freud, A. (1963). The concept of developmental lines. *Psychoanalytic Study of the Child, 18*, 245–265.

Freud, S. (1905a). Three essays on the theory of sexuality (1905). In James Strachey (Ed. and Trans.), *The Standard Edition of the Complete Psychological Works of Sigmund Freud* (Vol. VII, pp. 123–246). London: The Hogarth Press.

Freud, S. (1905b). Jokes and their relationship to the unconscious. In James Strachey (Ed. and Trans.), *The Standard Edition of the Complete Psychological Works of Sigmund Freud* (Vol VIII). London: The Hogarth Press.

Freud, S. (1924). The dissolution of the Oedipal complex. In James Strachey (Ed. and Trans.), *The Standard Edition of the Complete Psychological Works of Sigmund Freud* (Vol. XIX, pp. 171–180). London: The Hogarth Press.

Furman, E. (1980). Transference and externalization in latency. *Psychoanalytic Study of the Child, 35*, 267–284.

Gilmore, K. (2002). Diagnosis, dynamics and development: considerations in the psychoanalytic assessment of children with AD/HD. *Psychoanalytic Inquiries, 22*, 372–390.

Goldings, H. J. (1974). Jump-rope rhymes and the rhythm of latency development in girls. *Psychoanalytic Study of the Child, 29*, 431–450.

Goodman, G., Bartlett, R. C., & Stroh, M. (2013). Mothers' borderline features and children's disorganized attachment representations as predictors of children's externalizing behaviors. *Psychoanalytic Psychology, 30*, 16–36.

Harley, M. (1962). The role of the dream in the analysis of a latency child. *Journal of the American Psychoanalytic Association, 62*, 271–288.

Hartmann, H., Kris, E., & Loewenstein, R. M. (1949). Comments on the formation of psychic structure. *Psychoanalytic Study of the Child, 2*, 11–38.

Hartmann, H. & Loewenstein, R. M. (1962). Notes on the superego. *Psychoanalytic Study of the Child*, 17, 42–81.

Hoffman, L. (2007). Do children when we interpret their defenses against unwanted affects. *Psychoanalytic Study of the Child*, 62, 291–313.

Jemerin, J. M. (2004). Latency and the capacity to reflect on mental states. *Psychoanalytic Study of the Child*, 59, 211–239.

Kaplan, L. J. (1974). The concept of the family romance. *Psychoanalytic Review*, 61, 169–202.

Knight, R. (2005). The process of attachment and autonomy in latency: a longitudinal study of 10 children. *Psychoanalytic Study of the Child*, 60, 178–210.

Knight, R. (2011). Fragmentation, fluidity, and transformation: nonlinear development in middle childhood. *Psychoanalytic Psychology*, 65, 19–47.

Kochanska, G., & Knaack, A. (2003). Effortful control as a personality characteristic of young children: antecedents, correlates and consequences. *Journal of Personality*, 71, 1087–1112.

Kulish, N. (2002). Female sexuality: the pleasure of secrets and the secret of pleasure. *Psychoanalytic Study of the Child*, 57, 151–176.

Livingstone, S. (2003). Children's use of the internet: reflections on the emerging research agenda. *New Media & Society*, 5, 147–166.

Loewald, H. W. (1979). The waning of the oedipal complex. *Journal of the American Psychoanalytic Association*, 27, 751–775.

Loke, I. C., Heyman, G. P., & Gorgie, J. (2011). Children's moral evaluations of reporting the transgressions of peers: age differences in evaluation of tattling. *Developmental Psychology*, 47, 1757–1762.

Luna, B., Garver, K. E., Urban, T. A., Lazar, N. A., & Sweeney, J. A. (2004). Maturation of cognitive processes from late childhood to adulthood. *Child Development*, 75, 1357–1372.

Maccoby, E. (2002). Gender and group process: a developmental perspective. *Current Directions in Psychological Science*, 11, 54–58.

Main, M., Kaplan, N., & Cassidy, J. (1985). Security in infancy, childhood and adulthood: a move to the level of representation. *Monographs of the Society for Research in Child Development*, 50, 66–104.

Martin, C. L. & Ruble, D. (2004). Children's search for gender cues. *Current Directions in Psychological Science*, 13, 67–70.

Mahon, E. (1991). The dissolution of the Oedipus: a neglected cognitive factor. *Psychoanalytic Quarterly*, 60, 628–634.

Martin, C. L. & Ruble, D. (2004). Children's search for gender cues. *Current Directions in Psychological Science, 13*, 67–70.

McColgan, M. & Giardino, A. P. (2005). Internet poses multiple risks to children and adolescents. *Pediatric Annals, 34*, 405–414.

Nobes, G. & Pawson, C. (2003). Children's understanding of social rules and social status. *Merrill-Palmer Quarterly, 49*, 77–99.

Novick, K. K. & Novick, J. (1994). Postoedipal transformations: latency, adolescence and pathogenesis. *Journal of the American Psychoanalytic Association, 42*, 143–169.

Novick, K. K. & Novick, J. (1996). A developmental perspective on omnipotence. *Journal of Clinical Psychoanalysis, 5*, 129–173.

Novick, K. K. & Novick, J. (2004). The superego and the 2-system model. *Psychoanalytic Inquiry, 24*, 232–256.

Pedersen, S., Vitaro, F., Barker, E., & Borge, A. I. H. (2007). The timing of middle-childhood peer rejection and friendship: linking early behavior to early adolescent adjustment. *Child Development, 78*, 1037–1051.

Piaget, J. (1932). *The Moral Development of the Child*. New York: Harcourt.

Piaget, J. (1962). *Play, Dreams and Imitation in Childhood*. New York: Norton & Co.

Piaget, J. & Inhelder, B. (1969). *The Psychology of the Child*. New York: Basic Books.

Ponitz, C. C., McClelland, M. M., Matthews, S., & Morrison, F. J. (2009). A structured observation of behavioral self-regulation and its contribution to Kindergarten outcomes. *Developmental Psychology, 45*, 605–619.

Rothstein, A. (1998). Neuropsychological development and psychological conflict. *Psychoanalytic Quarterly, 67*, 218–234.

Sandler, J. & Freud, A. (1984). Discussions in the Hampstead Index in "The Ego and the Mechanisms of Defense": XII. The ego and the id at puberty. *Bulletin of the Anna Freud Centre, 7*, 5–14.

Sarnoff, C. A. (1971). Ego structure in latency. *Psychoanalytic Quarterly, 40*, 387–414.

Shapiro, T. (1976). Latency revisited—the age of 7 plus or minus 1. *Psychoanalytic Study of the Child, 31*, 79–105.

Solnit, A. J. (1998). Beyond play and playfulness. *Psychoanalytic Study of the Child, 53*, 102–110.

Sroufe, A. L., Bennett, C., Englund, M., Urban, J., & Shulman, S. (1993). The significance of gender boundaries in preadolescence:

contemporary correlates and antecedents of boundary violation and maintenance. *Child Development, 64*, 455–466.

Suizzo, M. (2000). The social-emotional and cultural contexts of cognitive development: neo-Piagetian perspectives. *Child Development, 71*, 846–849.

Weinstein, L. & Saul, L. (2005). Psychoanalysis as cognitive remediation: dynamic and Vygotskian perspectives in the analysis of an early adolescent dyslexic girl. *Psychoanalytic Study of the Child, 60*, 239–262.

Weinstein, L. & Shustorovich, E. (2011). Coherence, competence and confusion in narratives of middle childhood. *Psychoanalytic Study of the Child, 65*, 79–102.

6

Preadolescence and Early Adolescence: Introduction to the Adolescent Process and the Challenges of Sexual Maturation

Overview

A Brief History of Controversy

Controversies about adolescence as a developmental phase distinguished by turmoil have surrounded its study since the turn of the twentieth century, when it was formally introduced by American psychologist G. Stanley Hall with the publication of his two-volume tome: *Adolescence: Its Psychology and Its Relations to Physiology, and Anthropology, Sociology, Sex, Crime, Religion, and Education* (1904). In his preface, Hall put forth a resonant picture of adolescence as a transition full of "sturm und drang" in which the rupture of "old moorings" gradually achieved a "new birth" (1904, p. xiii). The assertion that turmoil was a universal feature of the bridge from childhood to adulthood was challenged in academic circles by the publication of Margaret Mead's study of Samoan society (1928/2001). She described the Samoan transition to adulthood as smooth and trouble-free, refuting Hall's arguments for inevitable biologically determined upheaval. Despite subsequent corrections of Mead's glowing portrayal in anthropological literature, the debate about adolescence continued in developmental and related disciplines, coalescing around two related questions: (1) is adolescence inevitably tumultuous? (A. Freud, 1958; Rutter et al., 1976); (2) is it a universal psychobiological process with recognizable features that transcend culture (Dasen, 2000)?

In regard to the second question, many developmental thinkers consider adolescence a "cultural invention" (Stone & Church, 1955), produced by extended schooling and dependence on parents (Schlegel & Barry, 1991). Blos, who devoted his professional life to the exploration of the adolescent process, implicitly endorsed this view with his statement: "Puberty is an act of nature and adolescence is an act of man" (Blos, 1979, p. 405). Certainly, the biological transformations of puberty are undeniable and its arrival is frequently marked by traditional societies with "coming of age" rituals. These detractors and others in related fields concur that puberty can leadto a sustained developmental process, primarily in settings where social circumstances demand adjustments, extensions, and disruptions of traditional sequences (Brown & Larson, 2002; Dasen, 2000). From this perspective, adolescence is an artifact of postindustrial, Western society in which the passage from childhood to adulthood is prolonged and chaotic. Sociologists implicate the loss of guidance provided by tradition and religion, expanded educational opportunities for both boys and girls, urbanization, and other social trends (Dasen, 2000) in disrupting child-to-adult-role continuity. In contrast, anthropologist supporters of universality contend that in *any* society, adolescence encompasses the "social stage intervening between childhood and adulthood in the passage through life" (Schlegel & Barry, 1991, p. 8) with its own activities and expectations, during which learning in preparation for adulthood takes place. But is it inevitably tumultuous?

That question has dogged the study of adolescence in the fields of developmental psychology and psychoanalysis. Hall's original description was embraced by many psychoanalytic thinkers, most notably Anna Freud, as a metaphor for the "interruption of peaceful growth" (A. Freud, 1958, p. 267) and inevitable turmoil of the adolescent transition (Wolf, Gedo, & Terman, 1972). From the viewpoint of Anna Freud and her followers, the universality of the process was based on the biological engine of sexual development, with the associated augmentation of drive, bodily transformation, resurgence of oedipal dynamics and consequent reconfiguration of the parent–child relationship—presumably a challenge for every adolescent regardless of culture. Some of the most renowned adolescent theorists who followed Anna Freud, such as Blos and especially Erikson, explicitly emphasized the shaping role of the environment and the impact of social forces on the process, but its biological inevitability and associated upheaval were not in dispute.

Arguments against the idea of turmoil arose almost immediately from American developmental researchers. Their studies, based on self-report and questionnaires, documented that the majority of adolescents and their parents acknowledged little distress or disruption (Bandura, 1964; Offer, 1965; Offer & Offer, 1968; Rutter et al., 1976). Offer, and Offer and Offer's findings, collected from large nonclinical samples, seemed to decisively disprove the idea of adolescent upheaval and led to its rejection within mainstream developmental theory and research for decades (Steinberg, 2000). Some of the discrepancy in the observations informing these divergent opinions has been attributed to the methodology and type of population surveyed. Psychoanalytic observers derived their ideas from clinical populations and access to a deeper level of experience. Even within psychoanalysis, there are still dissenters in regard to aspects of the classical theory. For example, Blos' extension of Mahler's separation–individuation model to describe the *second individuation* (see glossary) of adolescence is decried as a misrepresentation based on observations of psychopathology and a failure to consider the role of prior familial history. These commentators insist that the restructuring of the parent–child relationship proceeds with or without turmoil in accordance with the adolescent's childhood experience of attachment security (Doctors, 2000; Marohn, 1998). Renunciation, disruption, and ambivalence are products of insecure ties between parent and child.

However, the turn of the twenty-first century has witnessed a sea change within developmental science with the reinstatement of the phenomenon of adolescent turmoil. As one prominent developmental psychologist observed, the prevailing scientific view never really convinced the public anyway (Steinberg, 2000). Parents continued to struggle with adolescent children, and literature, movies, and other media continued to highlight their conflicts with the older generation, their existential angst in the search for identity, and their fraught peer relationships, in addition to their action orientation, sensation-seeking, and romance with danger and risk. New findings from family studies and the neuroscience of adolescence support the picture of adolescent turmoil held all along by parents and developmental psychoanalysts (Arnett, 1999). Radical transformations in the child's neural, neuroendocrine, physical, psychological, familial, and peer systems are the substrate for the "difficulties in the control of behavior and emotion" responsible for a 200% increase in morbidity and mortality of this age group compared with school-age children (Dahl, 2004, p. 3). This dramatic statistic is testament to the struggles of adolescents in our society. It is supported by family studies that highlight the uptick in conflict and disruption generated in families by the presence of an adolescent, which, of course, every parent knew all along (Garcia-Ruiz et al., 2013).

Duration and Subphases of Adolescence

Therefore, after a century of debate in related sciences, Hall's original assertion of storm and stress is in renaissance. Many of his other ideas presaged twenty-first century findings and trends, such as the importance of adolescent brain maturation, sensation-seeking, moodiness, and potential for criminal behavior (Arnett, 2006; Dahl & Hariri, 2005). In addition, his integration of multiple perspectives to create an inclusive picture of adolescent development anticipated contemporary multisystem theorizing. From our point of view, his timing of the process, occasionally noted but rarely addressed in the literature that followed (for an exception, see Arnett, 2000), is also forward-thinking and ahead of his time, especially as college attendance (*the psychosocial moratorium*—see glossary), often cited as the cause of extended adolescence, was less widespread, and pathways to adulthood were more highly structured at the turn of the twentieth century compared with today. Hall's timetable encompassed the period from 14 years old, then the average age of puberty (as determined by menarche), to age 24 when adult milestones were usually achieved. Remarkably, even Shakespeare alluded to the lengthiness of the adolescent process and its extension into the twenties; he also presciently recognized its stirrings at the very beginning of the second decade:

> I would that there were no age between ten and three and twenty, or that youth would sleep out the rest, for there's nothing in between but getting wenches with child, wronging the ancientry, stealing, fighting... (Winter's Tale, Act III)

Unfortunately, this comprehensive time frame did not become the norm in considerations of the adolescent process.

Indeed, adolescent timing and subphases have resisted systematization. Although onset at puberty is widely accepted, given the link to observable biological events, the early, middle, and late subdivisions are used inconsistently, creating some confusion as to the associated tasks and expectations, and the conclusion of adolescence is similarly unstandardized. The result is widely discrepant categorizations and findings and the rise of a new developmental phase, "emerging adulthood" (Arnett, 2000), touted as the twenty-first century equivalent to the twentieth century "discovery" of adolescence. Jeffery Arnett, the major proponent and theorist of this phase, places emerging adulthood between ages 18 and 24, thus ending adolescence at age 18. He justifies his choice on the basis of the earlier onset of puberty and the ubiquity of high school education in 2000 (95%) compared to Hall's day. Arnett asserts that the ages between 11 and 18 encompass contemporary adolescence, from the current age of puberty to the end of standardized educational experience. Other theorists suggest that today's trend toward earlier puberty, universal college attendance, and later achievement of the markers of adulthood have simply elongated the adolescent process at the expense of childhood and adulthood. These controversies have colored the delineation of early, middle, and late adolescence and the nature of associated developmental tasks. Such variability underscores the reality that adolescence, whose beginning is marked by biological events, has no comparable marker for its subphases or its end, despite the reality that these divisions continue to be meaningful to observers.

Adolescence in Context

In contrast to such blurred boundaries and their idiosyncratic designation in the literature, onset at puberty has been confidently presented as a sharp and decisive biological event. However, current views on the arrival of puberty note that it can occur at a range of points in the adolescent transformation; contemporary neuroscientists suggest that adolescence is more accurately understood as "series of soft events" (Spear, 2000) that begin in preadolescence and progress over the course of years. The singular psychological import of the first menstruation and nocturnal emission (traditionally considered pubertal markers) is undeniable, but puberty occurs in the context of an ongoing multisystemic transition already in progress. The tremendous intra- and interindividual variability in the sequence and pace of this soft process arises from the idiosyncratic maturation of myriad genetic, physiological and psychological systems. These in turn are powerfully affected by "socioecological factors" that influence the gamut, from the timing of puberty to the serial expectations of cognitive performance, behavior, and productivity maintained in a given society (Worthman, 1999). Cultural, microcultural, and extracultural environmental factors, which figure as lesser players in prior development, are increasingly important throughout adolescence and young adulthood. For example, environmental provision, in terms of socioeconomic class, medical care, and diet, outweighs genetic contributions in determining pubertal timing in contemporary postindustrial Western societies, now earlier by almost two years. Current nutritional state and anticipation of future adequate nutrition are fundamental to regulating the release of kisspeptins, identified in contemporary neuroscience as the "gatekeeper" of the hormonal–neural interaction responsible for the cascade of internal events and bodily changes resulting in the specific events of puberty and the widespread transformation of brain, sexual organs, and mental life (Spear, 2010). The concrete evidence of reproductive readiness, i.e. menarche, and first emission is vastly significant in its effect on the child's self-representation as a sexual and gendered person, but even these uniquely personal constructs are "contextualized" in regard to the surround. An individual sees his or her status in complex relationship to the peer group (Worthman, 1999, p. 136), family attitudes, and culture. Environmental factors—including socioeconomics, media input, peer trends, and educational opportunities, in addition to specific familial influences—exert a powerful influence on developmental progression, expectations, demands, and opportunities.

This applies to the intrapsychic experience of sexual development as well. The adolescent faces a marked upsurge of sexual and aggressive drives and the simultaneous evolution of his or her unique and idiosyncratic sexuality. The "central masturbation fantasy," a composite of the repressed oedipal constellation of childhood (Laufer, 1976) and its subsequent elaborations, gradually establishes the characteristic individual "sex-print;" that is, the unique narrative and requirements for arousal (Person, 1999). Masturbation in adolescence serves to integrate both the newly matured sexual body and this central fantasy into the self-representation. The task of young adolescents is to come to terms with their bodies and adapt their fantasies so that they find outlets for their desires beyond masturbatory activity (Shapiro, 2008). This process of "normalization" transforms fantasy—be it perverse, frightening, sadistic, masochistic, and/or forbidden by contemporary mores—into a form that has potential for real gratification. The conditions and constraints that are brought to bear on the reworking of fantasy are inevitably a byproduct of the peer culture embedded in an ambient society with its own cultural sex-print: What is allowed, with whom, when, and with what room for individual preferences—all these parameters and more are prescribed by the cultural surround. In contemporary Western post-postmodern culture, the powerful onslaught of sexual messages, the confusing official stance promoting abstinence, the media blitz of highly objectified and idealized body representations, the access to cyber-sex, such as pornography, virtual relationships, anonymous chat rooms, and so on, the ongoing heated discourse about traditional views of "normalcy" and "deviation," deliver complex messages to children on the threshold of their sexual lives (Corbett, 2013). These are more or less in contrast to individual family culture. Although there are families that embody contemporary sensibility, many do not. Adolescents whose sexual desires violate family constraints (including gay and lesbian youth) or their own moral code are often unable to feel "normal" despite the permissive culture. They feel deep shame, guilt, or self-hatred with lasting impact on their identity, object relations, mood, and narcissistic balance (Laufer, 1976; Laufer & Laufer, 1984).

Similarly, other key developmental arenas of this phase are shaped by context. Adolescent ego, cognitive, and affective expansion is the multifaceted product of maturation influenced by a context promoting or impeding these capacities. For example, burgeoning adolescent appreciation of adult "scripts" that encompass subtle and conflicting emotion is scaffolded by environmental exposure and direct instruction (Hauser & Smith, 1991). The evolution of the superego, a mental agency that undergoes multiple transitions during adolescence, is similarly reworked in context. The processes of externalization and reintegration are highly vulnerable to influence by the family, the peer group, and the larger culture upholding authoritarian, democratic, or other values (Blum, 1985). This is well illustrated by the radically different moral agendas and endorsed attitudes associated with generations; the values of the 1950s compared with the 1960s reflect social changes wrought by myriad factors and epitomized (and often driven) by the conformist or rebellious *youth culture* (see glossary) of the day. The current ascendance of *technoculture* (see glossary) poses a new challenge, as it offers unprecedented opportunities to express impulses that are magically sequestered from superego controls and external censure, as in violent gaming or cyberbullying (Turkel, 2007). This twenty-first century challenge to superego consolidation has yet to be fully understood.

Thus, even though we endorse the notion of adolescence as a universal developmental experience, we recognize that the overarching developmental themes reflect the active interface between the individual and society. Pubertal timing, body transformation, self-consciousness and egocentrism (Elkind & Bowen, 1979; Westen, 1990), focus on peers, emerging sexual orientation, sexual fantasy, access to sex and romantic relationships, pressure toward action and sensation, the twin tasks of individuation and evolution of personal identity, the emergence of personal values and ideals, extended education, the search for one's place in the world—all depend on the particular era and cultural context. There is little dispute about the increase in parent–child conflict, but it too is greatly affected by a multiplicity of factors ranging from ethnicity to personal attachment history (Garcia-Ruiz et al., 2013; Phinney et al., 1990).

Emerging Cognitive Capacities

In Piaget's scheme, adolescent mental capacities are distinguished by the emergence of *formal operations* (see glossary), which include advances in logical reasoning, deductive thinking, abstraction, and executive function. These developments have a far-reaching impact on academic performance, depth of understanding, and expertise, as well as the capacity to self-reflect and think about others. They introduce a new depth of questioning in regard to expectations and values transmitted by adults and society, and are essential to many tasks of adolescence: individuation, identity formation, intimate relationships, and the establishment of personal standards. Formal operations thus scaffold many developmental advances and shape adolescent sensibility and subjective experience. Intra-psychically, they bring major advances in self-reflection: thinking about one's own thoughts, reflecting on one's values, and recognizing one's past and future as belonging to oneself (Kuhn, 2008; Westen, 1990). At first disequilibrated by the bodily transformation and attempts to individuate from the close identification with parents and their views, the self-concept gradually gains depth and complexity, moving from self-description based on observable features (such as physical beauty or athleticism) to psychological ones, and providing a foundation for identity.

These novel thinking skills evolve in dynamic interaction with environmental nutriment and expectation. The appearance of new or matured cognitive capacities occurs in or out of sync with the evolving demands of the academic and social environment. As teenagers progress from middle school to high school to college in our society, executive function, higher level abstract thinking, and hypothetico-deductive reasoning (formal operations) are expected to come on line. Similarly, requirements for the related capacities to exercise judgment, apply moral reasoning, read social cues, mentalize empathically, weigh consequences, manage impulses, and self-regulate are built into the progression from dependence on parents to autonomous decision making and self-governance. Much adolescent existential angst, soul-searching, romantic yearnings, and "noble purpose" (Brooks, 2012) depend on the emergence of abstract thinking, perspective-taking, and independently determined ideals.

As always, emerging capacities do not appear in unison and fully evolved, nor are they stable, internally consistent, or fully realized in every arena. Writing about adolescence, Piaget observed that as the individual passes through cognitive development, the emergence of new capacities is both increasingly dependent on environmental stimulation and requires individual aptitude for a given subject (Piaget, 1972/2008) to produce the specialized intellectual capacity that characterizes adulthood. Even some "innate" cognitive capacities associated with formal operations and executive function can be cultivated by deliberate educational and experiential input (Carpandale & Lewis, 2004; Peskin & Wells-Jopling, 2012). Postsecondary school education thus promotes and consolidates the differentiation and specialization of selective arenas of cognition in late adolescence.

It is only in late adolescence or postadolescence that mature synthetic function is consistently operational. Synthetic function is a comprehensive emergent ego capacity, responsible for "psycho-synthesis" (Freud, 1919, p. 161); it facilitates the integration of cognition and emotion, and the development of coherent and meaningful life narratives, a mature time sense (Colarusso, 1988), and the final steps of identity, individuation, and superego consolidation. Synthetic function overlaps the description of executive function described in the neurocognitive developmental literature (Gilmore, 2002), but is broader in scope, affecting the complex process of consolidating of the adult personality organization—its characteristic defensive patterns, sublimatory channels, object relations, and superego function (Blos, 1968).

The variable appearance of these emerging capacities reflects the rapid but uneven changes in the brain that are the focus of current neuroscientific research. Recent findings suggest that adolescence is a time of remarkable neural plasticity, when the brain undergoes significant sculpting and remodeling primarily through neuronal pruning and enhanced connectivity. Many typical early and mid-adolescent tendencies, demonstrable in mammals and other species, have been correlated with this transformation, including the heightened focus on peer culture and interest in sensation seeking, both of which are speculated to serve the evolutionary goal of minimizing incestuous relations (Spear, 2004). The uneven progression of brain development is also considered a causal factor in the early adolescent's notorious disjunction between arousal, sensation-, and novelty-seeking on the one hand, and impulse control and regulatory capacities on the other. Neural remodeling continues into late adolescence through the twenties and is presumably a factor, in synergy with intrapsychic, environmental, and cultural forces, producing the shifting forms of adolescence at different stages in this process: "adolescence is, of its essence, a period of transitions rather than a moment of attainment" (Rosenblum, 1990, p. 63).

A Pragmatic Definition of Subphases

Our division of adolescence into three adolescent subphases is consistent with contemporary conventions of school progression and relates to the opportunities and requirements associated with them: early adolescence, 11 to 14 years, corresponding to middle school, mid adolescence, 14 to 18 years, roughly corresponding to high school and late adolescence, 18 to 24 years, to college. Of course, school shifts, entailing academic expectations, levels of social competence, and autonomous functioning, can be out of sync with the physical and psychological development of the child, but they constitute meaningful groupings in which environmental demand, a complex amalgam issuing from school, peers, family, and media (both social and commercial) impinges on individual psychology. As such, they are "normative-social shifts" that produce a remarkable degree of uniformity, mandated by a given culture in any given cohort (Hendry & Kloep, 2011). As during all adolescent phases, the ubiquitous peer group, augmented in today's world by the equally ubiquitous social media, is the pacesetter for biopsychosocial progression. Developing adolescents measure their success and accrue confidence as they conform to the yardstick established by the majority. Most children enter middle school, high school, and college exquisitely aware of how they compare with their peers and what is "expected" in terms of their bodies, their cognitive capacities, their life-experience, and their social competence.

Consistent with a modified view of phases as heuristically useful but interpenetrating, and grossly recognizable but variable within and between individuals, the tasks of adolescence are addressed in all subphases; some are more characteristic of one period or another but all are revisited over the course of the decade. Integration of the sexual and gendered body into the self-representation is an early challenge, whether the child is precocious, average, or delayed in pubertal development. Bodies are on the mind of the young teen; both physical attractiveness and pubertal status are powerful determinants in positioning him or her in the peer group. The relationship to the family is a potent arena of change, whether or not it is visibly disruptive, and the superego, as the parents' intrapsychic outpost, is deposed early in adolescence as a revered source of guidance and ego support. The superego undergoes a series of transformations, some of which can seem alien and lawless while in ascendance. Tasks such as individuation and identity formation cover the broad sweep of the adolescent process, taking the forefront in the adolescent's mental life at different junctures. For example, identity is a conscious preoccupation at various points: between high school and what follows—college or employment—and again at the confrontation with "the rest of your life" triggered by college graduation or the sense of settling into a career "for life," but the process of identity formation is continuous. Achievement of individuation and the progression of identity formation facilitate personality consolidation and synthesis that mark the final steps toward adulthood and scaffold the capacity to commit to a love object, a career, and a self-representation that signifies satisfactory resolution. As we discuss in chapter 8, this process has extended up to age 30 in Western postindustrial society, leading to the proposal of a new subphase, emerging adulthood.

Overview of Preadolescence

The child's entry into preadolescence, which spans the years between 10 and the onset of puberty, brings the relative stability of latency to a close. The bodily transformations of this phase are less profound than those of adolescence proper, but the child nonetheless undergoes a complex psychological adjustment to the subjective sense of increased hormonal production, as well as to more tangible increases in skeletal growth, body fat, and physical prowess. Moreover, the emergence of secondary sexual characteristics—such as breast budding for girls, typically at 10.5, and testicular growth for boys, at around 11—irreversibly alters the familiar contours of the latency body and foreshadows the attainment of full sexual maturity (Brooks-Gunn & Warren, 1988; Paikoff & Brooks-Gunn, 1991). Indeed, preadolescent children are remarkably adept at discerning their peers' progression toward puberty and are highly reactive to perceptions that they are out of step with age-mates (Brooks-Gunn & Warren, 1988; Mendle et al., 2010). Preadolescence merits recognition as a distinct, albeit brief period in development because of these features: increased drive toward autonomy and separation, sense of internal disequilibrium, and premonitory signs of rupture in the parent–child relationship, combined with the early indications of the pubertal "cascade" of physiological changes (Blos, 1958; Knight, 2005, 2011).

The classic psychoanalytic view of this phase focuses on the quantitative increase in preadolescent sexual drive, which, after a prolonged state of relative dormancy in latency, brings a recrudescence of earlier psychosexuality. Under the pressure of intensified sexual feelings, oedipal wishes are revived. The threat of oedipal strivings leads to a defensive resurgence of pregenitality, accompanied by the child's fears of re-engulfment in the infantile mother–child relationship (Blos, 1958). Behaviorally, these processes are exemplified through the preadolescent's familiar increased motoric restlessness, oppositionality, rejections of maternal closeness, and manifestations of oral greed and anality. A prior consolidation of latency capacities is considered the major prerequisite for handling intensified sexual and aggressive impulses and for tolerating regressive trends.

Both girls and boys are subject to similar internal pressures and regressions, but a number of theorists elaborate sex-specific pathways through this developmental period. Blos views boys' increase in castration anxiety, specifically linked to preoedipal fantasies of attack by the phallic mother, as the universal hallmark of male entry into preadolescence. Renewed castration fears are fueled by the boy's very tangible experience of increased growth and sensitivity of the penis and testes, as well as by the environmental reality of an earlier height spurt in female agemates (Bell, 1965; Blos, 1958). The prepubertal boy's resulting fear and envy of girls propels him decisively toward same-sex peers and the perceived safety of male groups. Girls' chief anxieties involve re-enmeshment with and passive surrender to the mother. They tend to seek relief not only via dyadic female friendships, but also through premature flight toward heterosexual contact (Blos, 1958; Dahl, 1993; Fisher, 1991). Transient, superficial but intensely intimate girl pairs are common, involving concrete identification and experimentation with each other's demeanor and opinions (Fisher, 1991). Both sexes pursue increasing distance from the maternal object, who is consciously experienced as overbearing and intrusive.

The body's inevitable progression toward puberty signals the encroachment of gender definition and finality. In the classic psychoanalytic literature, acceptance of one's sex and renouncing bisexuality or gender fluidity are dominant psychological tasks of this phase. For girls, preadolescence is often a unique period of fluctuation between male and female identifications. Rapid, dramatic changes in demeanor, for example, from tomboyish attire to precocious glamour, are common (Dalsimer, 1979; Fisher, 1991). Contemporary thinkers have suggested that girls' gender fluidity is better tolerated in Western society than boys'. In one study, around half of women and girls reported a preadolescent tendency toward conventionally boyish behaviors, such as sports or affinities for "male" toys, which receded as puberty approached (McHale et al., 2004). Environmental intolerance may play a significant role in boys' considerably greater behavioral gender conformity (Friedman 2001; Galatzer-Levy & Cohler, 2002).

The preadolescent's shift toward autonomy and beginning resistance to parental control augur the unraveling of infantile object ties during early and middle adolescence, engendering feelings of deep loss and insecurity (Knight, 2005, 2011). In part, closer connection to peers satisfies object longing and compensates for increasing disillusionment with the parents (A. Freud, 1949). Moreover, the preadolescent's capacity for relational complexity is enhanced by the onset of formal operational thinking. The child's development toward increasingly intimate bonds was described by Sullivan (1953) as the "quiet miracle" of this phase. The child's sense of self and others acquires abstract psychological dimensionality, which facilitates mentalization and promotes an interest in peers' emotional qualities. A yearning for mutual intimacy, in the form of reciprocal understanding and jointly held perspectives, replaces the latency child's focus on friendship as a venue for shared games and activities (Auerbach & Blatt, 1996; Buhrmester, 1990). The capacity for greater social complexity helps the preadolescent navigate the demands of this age group as he or she emerges from the rigid, peer-enforced sex-linked boundaries and divisions of the latency phase. Preteens must find ways to integrate powerful peer group standards and sanctions with dawning interest and excitement in the sex to which they are increasingly attracted (Sroufe et al., 1993).

Overview of Early Adolescence

Preadolescence is thus the launching pad for the massive acceleration of growth and reconfiguration of the body that gathers steam until the physical self has morphed into a powerful, sexed, sexual, and reproductively functional body. Whether this transformation is achieved in months or years, whether it feels interminable or sudden, it is "body drama" in the subjective experience of the adolescent (Redd, 2007). Mastering and owning the changing sexual and gendered body continue to absorb and challenge the mind throughout the early phase of adolescence (Laufer & Laufer, 1984). The accompanying surge of sexual and aggressive impulses creates internal pressure toward action. The preadolescent disengagement from parents is now augmented by the need to define the self in the world, have experience, and seek new outlets for excitement and urgenct desires.

The idealized paradigm of childhood, exemplified by a self-representation as an innocent embedded in the familial embrace, sharing values, and accepting the subordinate role is dissolved by the reality of a sexually equipped body with a growing set of adult capacities and a powerful need to seek outlets. Family relationships fray (Steinberg, 2000) as parental authority comes under scrutiny and loses its sovereignty. The close correspondence between the latency superego and the parental voice is shaken, and the peer group rises in importance as the standard bearers for behavior. The typical peer hierarchy of early adolescence is cliquish, exclusionary, and cruel, but holds sway as the barometer of what is desirable, cool, and "popular." Indeed, peer connection and acceptance have been empirically correlated with favorable social, emotional, and academic adjustment during adolescence, while peer rejection is linked to low mood and delinquency (Bagwell et al., 2000). As the middle school experience gradually redefines the child's social life, cliques achieve heightened power and importance. Although these groups threaten the child with enormous anxiety about exclusion, they simultaneously serve as highly influential and increasingly common sources of socialization. The entry into middle school, in fifth or sixth grade, initiates the young teen into a changed world: a sudden decline in teacher support, a dizzying array of choices and academic classes, and exposure to the potentially risky behavior of older teens (Molloy, Ram, & Gest, 2011). The early teenager's successful adjustment to its culture and academics is foundational to later adolescent school achievement.

The predilection to action, sensation- and novelty-seeking, impulsivity, and group contagion are most typically realized under conditions of high arousal created by drives pressing for release and by the need to maintain status and connection among like-minded peers (Steinberg, 2004). The confluence of these factors can plunge the early adolescent into the array of risky behaviors favored by the contemporaneous group and amply illustrated by older teens, including use of illegal substances and body injury, both accidental and purposeful (such as cutting and today's "salt and ice challenge"), dangerous violations of laws and rules, unprotected sexual activity, cyber-bullying, anonymous encounters in virtual reality, and so on. In addition, psychiatric disorders and addictions have their early roots in this phase, incubating until their diagnosable appearance in later adolescence.

The Body

Consistent with the "soft emergence" of pubertal changes, the bodily transformation usually begins in preadolescence, unfolding in a variable sequence. Typically the first indication for boys and girls alike is physical evidence of gonadarche (testicular enlargement for boys and breast budding for girls); adrenarche (pubic and body hair development) usually follows. The prior relatively flat growth curves for height and weight and the relatively good control over masturbation during latency foster a stable sense of bodily self. In the course of pubertal development, growth velocity gradually accelerates and reaches its peak, on average two years earlier for girls than for boys (Carswell & Stafford, 2008). As noted, the signal events of puberty—first menses and the first emission—are symbolic markers of the many biological transitions that characterize the adolescent process (Spear, 2000). The onset of pubertal development is significantly earlier than 25 years ago, but the age at full completion remains roughly the same, creating a more prolonged process of physical development than that experienced by the parent generation (Carswell & Stafford, 2008).

Thus the so-called "pubertal events" occur with considerable variability, somewhere in the sequence of bodily changes. Despite the multiplicity of the pubertal process, the sharp onset of menses and the first emission have huge intrapsychic impact on both boys and girls, because it unequivocally announces that adult sexuality and reproductive capacity have arrived. Although sexual bodies and privileges played a central role in the fantasies of the oedipal period, their advent was safely relegated to promises about the future, as consolation for the painful renunciation of oedipal strivings. The newly endowed sexual bodies and the ability to make babies are concrete evidence of entry into the adult world (Loewald, 1979, 1985), destabilizing the safely bounded and orderly familial hierarchy. This disequilibrium figures in an array of feelings and actions, from defiance of parental constraints to disavowal of the new maturational developments and determination to stay a child. The simultaneous shame, anxiety, and excitement of the pubertal moment attests to its psychological meaning as definitive evidence of the (nonetheless still wobbly) transformation into a sexual and gendered person in the minds of the child, family, and peer group.

The actual body is itself a formidable developmental challenge. Rapid physical growth, augmented sleep requirements, the emergence of secondary sexual characteristics, and the simultaneous need for and loss of control are powerful organizers for young teens who must integrate the new body and its functions into the self-representation and activities of daily life. The deep self-consciousness of early teen years arises in large part from the associated feelings of shame as the body transforms into an object—replete with odor, acne, menstrual accidents, and spontaneous erections—that requires attention and a set of new skills to avoid humiliating exposure. Moreover, this same body with all its embarrassing potential, may come to be objectified in a variety of contexts: as a "sex object" that elicits wanted and unwanted sexual responses from others, including adults; as an object to be measured against the barrage of beauty standards emanating from the media and the peer group (especially via social networking) (Vandenbosch & Eggermont, 2012); and by extension, as an object conferring status and popularity in the peer group or alternatively delivering disappointment, dashed hopes, and impediments to happiness. Overall appearance relative to peers and current media standards of "what's hot" are a source of gratification or anguish for young teens. The social hierarchy and cliques of middle school are often directly related to features such as attractiveness, physical prowess, and, of course, the appropriate developmental status, neither too early nor too late as dictated by the cohort. In fact, the impact of timing is highly significant for mental health in boys and girls (Kaltiala-Heino, Kosunen, & Rimpela, 2003): Pubertal development that noticeably precedes the peer group has long been documented as a handicap for girls, predisposing them to a host of psychosocial problems including depression, suicidality, anxiety, eating disorders, and poor academic performance (Mendle, Turkheimer, & Emery, 2007). In contrast, early timing was viewed as an asset for boys until recently, when accumulated evidence confirms its similar deleterious impact on male development (Mendle & Ferraro, 2012). Researchers suggest that the "maturational disparity" (Mendle & Ferraro, 2012, p. 50) in a physically developed but psychologically immature early adolescent is responsible for this robust finding of early development's negative impact Depression, suicidality, anxiety, disordered eating, delinquency, poor academic performance are all more prevalent in this group (Mendle & Ferraro, 2012, p. 58). So-called late bloomers, often a subjectively determined designation, are also susceptible to negative self-image and depression. No doubt the difficult transition into middle school is heightened by the developmental rise in self-consciousness in regard to one's own pubertal status and visible evidence of secondary sexual character-istics (Elkind, 1967).

The body is thus a fount of developmental demands for early adolescents. Many psychoanalytic writers specify that "ownership of the sexual body" is the preeminent challenge of this stage (Laufer & Laufer, 1984). Under the onslaught of sexual and aggressive drives, the superego, even though modified and liberalized over the course of latency, is unprepared. The ego's reliance on this bastion of paren-tal authority is disrupted. The former rules and simplified moral-ity of the superego cannot be reconciled with the excitement and temptation that suddenly are everywhere. The early adolescent ego becomes estranged from the prior "subjugated" latency self and latency superego, especially as the latter represents an internaliza-tion of the parental voice that forbids sexuality and aggression in the child or, at the very least, banishes it from view (Fonagy, 2008; Jacobson, 1961). Two characteristic but potentially problematic defensive organizations directed against the drives were described by Anna Freud in 1958: the "ascetic" adolescent, who disavows all bodily needs and the "uncompromising" adolescent, who resists any and all interference with the free expression of impulses. Modified versions of these defenses contribute to a variety of teen-age phenomena; for example, the girl with restricting anorexia who over-exercises or the boy who relentlessly seeks body modifications such as piercings and tattoos, drinks from his parents' liquor cabi-net, and obsessively plays violent games, in defiance of parental prohibition. In both examples, the body can become the concrete battleground for ownership. When these defenses dominate the personality organization, they interfere with the integration of the sexual body, sexual desire, and modulated aggression into an adap-tive self-representation.

The Family, Early Individuation, and Identity

As the body becomes more decisively sexed and sexual, parents and/ or their adolescent children feel uncomfortable with the level of physical affection that characterized their interactions in the past. The generational divide that reinforced the parental role and adult sexual prerogatives is blurred, The child is not a dependent little boy or girl, but a fully functional, sexually equipped young man or woman. Parents no longer represent unattainable adulthood with privileged access to sexual rights and moral authority (Levy-Warren, 2008). The powerful increment in sexual and aggressive drives in the incestuous setting of the family mobilizes defenses not only against impulses themselves, as in the ascetic or uncompromising defenses described in the preceding, but also vis-à-vis the objects of desire. Katan suggested the term *object removal* (1951) (see glossary) to describe a specific normative defense of early adolescence whereby the excitement of burgeoning sexuality is directed outside the family, resulting in a decisive turn away from the infantile objects toward the peer group.

Blos (1967) proposed the term second individuation, based on Mahler's separation–individuation paradigm, to conceptualize the adolescent's changing relationship with parents and its reverberations in mental structure. Before puberty, the primary infantile objects functioned as ego supports and, via identification, shaped the superego and reinforced the repression of the oedipal constellation. Even the apparently self-regulated late latency child selectively relies on parents as an auxiliary ego (Blos, 1967, p. 164). In Blos's formulation (1967), the process of individuation begins in early adolescence, as a result of the confluence of developmental events including the pressure of incestuous anxiety and alienation from the childhood self and superego. Sexual development, advances in ego capacities, and growing interest in the peer group promote the early adolescent's resistance to dependency on parents and heighten strivings for autonomy, agency, and self-determined values and goals. The prevailing family culture, including dictates or presumptions about gender role, sexuality, aggression, race, religion, politics, and ethnicity becomes subject to reconsideration as the young teenager strives to differentiate (Besser & Blatt, 2007). Parental authority is questioned and parental flaws become painfully obvious. The familiar reliance on parents and internalized parental injunctions is no longer an easy defensive strategy at the threshold of the wild world of teen activities, but without their support (in the form of moral guidance, performance valuation, or management of daily routines), the young adolescent ego, already buffeted from within by the drives, is weakened.

The need to establish a sense of psychic separation from parents contributes to many features of early adolescence. Conflicts with parents reach peak frequency in early adolescence, as distinguished from the peak intensity that occurs in mid-adolescence, encompassing chores and duties, annoying behaviors, and parental encroachment on privacy and autonomy (Laursen, Coy, & Collins, 1998). Interestingly, the type of conflict that emerges between parents and early adolescents is laden with gender messages; statistically, parents nag more about their sons' homework and grades in contrast to power struggles around their daughters' attire, independence, and socialization. This is especially the case between mothers and daughters (Allison & Schultz, 2004).

In general, early adolescent parent–child conflicts are generated by anxieties shared by both parents and children—about the upsurge of sexual and aggressive impulses, the increase in risky behaviors, and the simultaneous waning parental control. For young teens, arguing provides the opportunity to vent frustration and bolster their resistance against the regressive pull to childlike dependency and incestuous longings. Parents use the convenient vehicles of asserting discipline and demanding compliance with chores to allay their own anxieties and exert control over the potential misadventures of their bucking teens. Chronic bickering and arguments contribute to the ubiquitous adolescent feelings of alienation and existential loneliness that accompany the second individuation. The young adolescent turns away from parents and adults in general, channels desire, aggression, and rivalry into the peer group, and embraces the values of "youth culture" (see glossary). Inevitably, these developments create a significant obstacle to treatment in this age group.

Blos's conceptualization of the second individuation has been criticized for its emphasis on drive, the recrudescence of the oedipal constellation, and the assumption that a violent rupture of the internal parent–child bond is required, inevitably producing "adolescent turmoil." In an argument recalling a similar critique of Mahler's idea of rapprochement (Lyons-Ruth, 1991), self-psychologists and some attachment theorists suggest it is only insecurely attached children who create upheaval. Among securely attached children, strong internal attachment bonds to parents are lifelong and steadily maintained throughout adolescence (Doctors, 2000; Marohn, 1999). However, Blos was careful to point out that overtly defiant and parent-rejecting adolescents are likely to be sidestepping the individuation process, a more arduous and subtle realignment that does not require overt rebellion against parents, even while their idealization and sovereignty gradually declines. In our view, the concept of the second individuation, if broadened to include multiple systems such as cognitive development, self-representation, cultural trends, adolescent brain development, family relationships, and peer influences, is fundamental for adolescent development. Furthermore, as clarified by Kernberg (2006) and others (such as Koepke & Denissen, 2012), the "second individuation" and Erikson's "adolescent identity crisis" are fundamentally intertwined. The latter is the "normal symptomatic manifestation" of the individuation process (Kernberg, 2006, p. 972) and a key factor in its resolution. It is thus the intrapsychic partner in the process of identity formation taking place in relation to the environment.

The Peer Group

Individuation propels the young adolescent into a new consideration of whom he or she is in the eyes of the peer world and how he or she fits into the larger youth culture. The individual child's identity is subject to revision as the peer hierarchy assumes dominance. Despite the anxiety and self-doubt that the peer group can invoke, the complex web of peer friendships, cliques, and romances in middle school eclipse the importance of family and school input and have the potential to shatter self-representations supported by adults. The peer group is the barometer, the moral compass, and the pacesetter. It is the prism through which popular media trends, youth culture (Arnett, 2004), and standards in beauty, fashion, and body type are refracted.

The notion of the "imaginary audience" was proposed by Elkind (1967) to capture the young adolescent's egocentric preoccupation with how he or she is seen by others. Elkind hypothesized that the uptick in egocentrism observed in this age group reflected a glitch in the early stages of formal operational thinking. Research into this concept and its origins favored a different explanation of the manifest phenomenon. The early adolescent peer group actually does wield enormous power and deeply influences the teen, because it replaces the childhood idealization of parents and is now the primary source of personal affirmation (Furman & Buhrmester, 1992). This is no "imaginary" audience; it is very real, and its lasting impact on self-image is deeply chiseled into the adult personality organization (Blum, 1985). The early adolescent's self-consciousness and bodily concerns are often amplified by being out of step with the adolescent subculture, owing to physical, ethnic, interpersonal or other attributes that violate the prioritization of sameness (Laursen et al., 2010). Most children, including those with apparently solid peer connections, experience a drop in confidence at the point of entry into middle school (Eder & Kinney, 1995).

Middle school society is politically more complex and rigidly hierarchical, and can either cement or, less likely, transform "reputations" that were set by the peer group of grade school (Arnett, 2004, p. 259). Children who were popular or unpopular in grade school are, with rare exceptions, gathered into new versions of popular or unpopular cliques that are consensually validated and self-reinforcing. Despite the capacity for more nuanced and in-depth evaluation of others, such assessments matter very little in early middle school. Popularity is based on relatively superficial attributes with broad media endorsement such as athletic success, cheerleading, physical attractiveness, and ownership of brand name items; neither personality appeal nor academic success determines membership in the coveted clique (Garner et al., 2006). The values of the peer culture trump the values represented by school, parents, or even the professed personal preferences of a given individual.

Aggression of various types is more evident between students, undeterred by institutional policy. Indeed, relational aggression and bullying are everyday occurrences. Interestingly, studies of clique formation demonstrate that membership within cliques, especially those at extremes of popularity or unpopularity, does not reduce the risk of aggression, which is used for purposes of maintaining the pecking order. Indeed, qualities of popular, mid-level and unpopular cliques support the stereotypic portrayal of the mid-level cliques as generally kinder and more egalitarian, despite the popular cliques perceived attractiveness (Closson, 2009).

Social media has added another layer to middle school experience and adolescent identity formation. Facebook, Instagram, tumblr, kik, ask.fm, Twitter, and Snapchat are open to children 13 and up, but many of them are accessible to even younger, tech-savvy pradolescents or "tweens." Facebook and Twitter, which are well monitored and policed, have declined in popularity and "coolness," whereas other, newer sites are rapidly gaining users (estimated for ask.fm between 57 and 65 million users worldwide; Edwards, 2013; Van Grove, 2013). The potential dangers of these sites, which provide opportunities for teens to air crushes, spread gossip, bully others with complete anonymity, and observe the "dramas" of their peers, is frequently in the news, depicted as a deadly playground in which users drive each other to suicide.[1]

Social success in middle school has lasting impact on self-representation, reflecting the importance of this developmental portal. Despite personal incompatibility, dislike, and sometimes fear in regard to "popular kids," the middle schooler feels the weight of the values they seem to represent. Some children find reassurance and companionship in their membership in the self-described "unpopular" group, hoping that high school will liberate them from social stratification that seems set in stone. But even with that release, the impact of the middle school identity, as experienced within and reinforced by the peer group, has remarkable staying power intrapsychically and is often deeply engraved into adult personality (Jacobs, 2000).

Risk Behaviors and Early Evidence of Psychopathology

The emergence of a predilection toward risky behavior begins in early adolescence, evolving over the next decade or more, depending on the individual and the type of behavior. Risk behavior has been persuasively linked to the converging impact of asynchronous neural remodeling with resulting heightened impulsivity and novelty-seeking (Chambers et al., 2003), flight toward the peer group, heightened susceptibility to peer influence (Steinberg, 2000), and urges to engage with the real world through action (Chused, 1990). The desire to assert ownership of the body, in combination with peer group influence, impulsivity, and the urgent wish to *experience*, can lead to a range of body modifications (tattoos, piercings, and so on) and death-defying thrill-seeking. These behaviors reflect adolescents' determination to flout parental precautions (Altman, 2007) and assert their belief in their own invulnerability. Many chemical and nonchemical addictive behaviors, such as drinking, smoking, marijuana use, internet abuse (gambling, gaming, pornography, obsessive social media involvement), begin in the early teens and tend to augment in prevalence and severity over the course of early and mid-adolescence (Wills et al., 2004). Problem behavior theorists propose a risk-protective factors model that underscores the interaction of multiple systems both within and surrounding the adolescent, including, for example, prior psychological disturbance and absence of role models as negative factors and strong family bonds and neighborhood resources as protective ones (Jessor, 1977, 1991). These create a "web of causation" (Jessor, 1991, p. 601), increasing the likelihood of risk behaviors.

Age 14 is the peak age of onset of mental health disorders, including eating disorders ranging from widely prevalent partial to full-blown anorexia and/or bulimia, mood and anxiety disorders, psychosis, self-injurious behaviors, substance abuse, suicidality, and emerging personality disorders (Paus, Keshaven, & Giedd, 2008). A review of contemporary understanding of the typical changes in the brain during adolescence suggests that at least one of these disorders, namely schizophrenia, is "an exaggeration of typical adolescent changes" in the brain (Paus et al., 2008, p. 952) and that predispositions to addiction, a range of anxiety and mood disorders, and impulsivity have a basis in the pattern of neural alteration occurring over the course of adolescent development.

Summary

Adolescence is a transformative process that extends over the whole second decade of life and into the third. After the "juvenile pause" produced by neuronal inhibition of circulating hormones in middle childhood, a series of neuroendocrine interactions initiate a cascade of physiological changes that ultimately result in sexual and reproductive maturity. Even before the highly meaning-laden "events" of puberty, the preadolescent experiences a growth spurt in height (peaking at age 11 in girls and 13 in boys) and premonitory bodily changes. Only infancy compares in terms of the velocity of physical growth, involving gains of up to 12 inches in boys and 11.5 inches in girls between 10 and 18 years of age (August & Abbassi, 1998). Of course, gains in height are only one component in the physical transformation, which includes increase in circulating hormones (Grumbach, 2002), growth of secondary sexual characteristics, weight gain of more than 40 pounds (18.5 kg, of which 68% is fat-free mass) in girls and 60 pounds (30 kg, of which 82% is fat-free mass) in boys (Wei & Gregory, 2009), evidence of reproductive competence, and massive brain remodeling associated with emergence of higher level cognitive capacities. These changes create a profound challenge in mental life: self-representation, relationship to the body, individuation and evolution of independent identity, new capacities for sex, love, and romance, the development of abiding interests, and internally determined moral standards, ambitions, and life goals are the gradually accumulated achievements needed for the major decisions of adulthood.

Pre- and early adolescence mark the threshold and the first steps into the process. These introductory phases, encompassing roughly ages 10 to 14, are associated with peak growth velocity, development of secondary sex characteristics, evidence of reproductive competence, and initiation of the process of individuation. The latter is an intrapsychic process that evolves over the course of adolescence; it is essential for identity development and responsible adulthood. The major tasks of these phases include an important shift of focus from parents to peer group. Not yet in full command of an internal moral compass or brain-based regulatory capacities, early individuation from parents and the reduced oversight at school leaves the teen alone to wrestle with mounting pressure toward sensation-seeking, action, heightened sexual and aggressive impulses, a newly powerful and sexual body, and a domineering peer culture. Sensation-seeking and reward salience are on the rise, peaking at the transition from early to mid-adolescence and from middle school to high school (age 15), long before the self-regulation of late adolescence has developed (Steinberg, 2008). The early steps in adolescent transformation are deeply psychologically challenging not only for their own sake but because young teenagers are increasingly conscious of what lies ahead. Key points of pre- and early adolescence include the following:

- The early phases of adolescence are a time of bodily transformation, defensive distancing from parents, and vastly increased investment in the peer group. Preoccupation with body image and peer group status are common. Bullying and peer coercion are among the heightened social risks that the young adolescent, who is far less able and willing to seek parental help, must navigate alone. Preadolescence, from 10 years until the advent of puberty, is characterized by prodromal bodily changes, a subjective sense of inner disequilibrium, and an increased drive toward autonomy, which may take the form of parent–child conflict.
- Early adolescence, from 11 or 12 to 14 years, is marked by the arrival of pubertal events that contribute to a more

pronounced turn away from parents, increased domination of the peer group, and augmented pressure for sensation seeking and action.

- Psychiatric concerns for this age group include the onset of depression and eating disorders, along with an increase in self-injurious and risky behaviors.

Notes

1. From *Business Insider*: Users on this web site have successfully driven nine teenagers to kill themselves (Edwards, September 16, 2013).

References

Allison, B. N., & Schultz, J. B. (2004). Parent-adolescent conflict in early adolescence. *Adolescence*, *39*, 101–119.

Altman, N. (2007). The children of the children of the sixties. *Journal of Child and Adolescent Psychotherapy*, *6*, 5–23.

Arnett, J. J. (1999). Adolescent storm and stress reconsidered. *American Psychologist, 54*, 317–326.

Arnett, J.J. (2000). Emerging adulthood: a theory of development from the late teens through the twenties. *American Psychologist 55*, 469–480.

Arnett, J. J. (2004). *Adolescence and Emerging Adulthood: A Cultural Approach* (2nd ed.). Boston: Prentice Hall.

Arnett, J. J. (2006). G. Stanley Hall's *Adolescence*: Brilliance and nonsense. *History of Psychology*, *9*, 186–197.

Auerbach, J. S. & Blatt, S. J. (1996). Self-representation in severe psychopathology: the role of reflexive self-awareness. *Psychoanalytic Psychology*, *13*, 297–341.

August, G. P. & Abbassi, V. (1998). Growth and normal puberty. *Pediatrics*, *102*(s), 507–511.

Bagwell, C. L., Cole, J. D., Terry, R. A., & Lochman, J. E. (2000). Peer clique participation and social status in preadolescence. *Merrill-Palmer Quarterly*, *46*, 280–305.

Bandura, A. (1964). The stormy decade: fact or fiction? *Psychology in the Schools*, *1*, 224–231.

Bell, A. I. (1965). The significance of scrotal sac and testicles for the prepuberty male. *Psychoanalytic Quarterly, 34,* 182–206.

Besser, A. & Blatt, S. J. (2007). Identity consolidation and internalizing and externalizing problem behaviors in early adolescence. *Psychoanalytic Psychology, 24,* 126–149.

Blos, P. (1958). Preadolescent drive organization. *Journal of the American Psychoanalytic Association, 6,* 47–56.

Blos, P. (1967). The second individuation process in adolescence. *Psychoanalytic Study of the Child, 22,* 162–186.

Blos, P. (1968). Character formation in adolescence. *Psychoanalytic Study of the Child, 23,* 245–263.

Blos, P. (1979). *The Adolescent Passage: Developmental Issues.* New York: International Universities Press.

Blum, H. (1985). Superego formation, adolescent transformation, and the adult neurosis. *Journal of the American Psychoanalytic Association, 33,* 887–909.

Brooks, K. C. B. (2012). A grounded theory of the development of noble youth purpose. *Journal of Adolescent Research, 27,* 78–109.

Brooks-Gunn, J. & Warren, M. P. (1988). The psychological significance of secondary sexual characteristics in 9-11 year old girls. *Child Development, 59,* 1061–1069.

Brown, B. B., & Larson, R. W. (2002). The kaleidoscope of adolescence: experiences of the world's youth at the beginning of the 21st century. In B. B. Brown, W. L. Reed, & T. S. Saraswathi (Eds.), *World's youth: Adolescence in Eight Regions of the World* (pp. 1–20). Cambridge, UK: Cambridge University Press.

Buhrmester, D. (1990). Intimacy of friendship, interpersonal competence and adjustment during preadolescence and adolescence. *Child Development, 61,* 1101–1111.

Carpandale, J. I. M. & Lewis, C. (2004). Constructing an understanding of mind: the development of children's social understanding within social interaction. *Brain and Behavioral Sciences, 27,* 59–151.

Carswell, J. M. & Stafford, D. E. J. (2008). Normal physical growth and development. In L. Nienstein (Ed.), *Adolescent Health Care: A Practical Guide* (5th ed., pp. 3–26). Philadelphia: Lippincott Williams & Wilkins.

Chambers, R. A., Taylor, J. R., & Potenza, M. N. (2003). Developmental neurocircuitry of motivation in adolescence: a critical period of addiction vulnerability. *American Journal of Psychiatry, 160,* 1041–1052.

Chused, J. (1990). Neutrality in the analysis of action-prone adolescents. *Journal of the American Psychoanalytic Association, 38,* 679–704.

Closson, L. M. (2009). Aggressive and prosocial behaviors with early adolescent friendship cliques. What's status got to do with it? *Merrill-Palmer Quarterly, 55,* 406–435.

Colarusso, C. A. (1988). The development of time sense in adolescence. *The Psychoanalytic Study of the Child, 43,* 179–197.

Corbett, K. (2013). Shifting sexual cultures, the potential space of online relations and the promise of psychoanalytic listening. *Journal of the American Psychoanalytic Association, 61,* 25–44.

Dahl, E. K. (1993). The impact of divorce on a preadolescent girl. *Psychoanalytic Study of the Child, 48,* 193–207.

Dahl, R. E. (2004). Adolescent brain development: a period of vulnerabilities and opportunities. Keynote address. *Annals of the New York Academy of Science, 1012,* 1–22.

Dahl, R. & Hariri, A. R. (2005). Lessons from G. Stanley Hall: Connecting new research in biological sciences to the study of adolescent development. *Journal of Research in Adolescence, 15,* 367–382.

Dalsimer, K. (1979). From preadolescent tomboy to early adolescent girl—an analysis of Carson McCuller's *The Member of the Wedding. Psychoanalytic Study of the Child, 34,* 445–461.

Dasen, P. R. (2000). Rapid social change and the turmoil of adolescence: a cross-cultural perspective. *International Journal of Group Tensions, 29,* 17–49.

Doctors, S. (2000). Attachment-individuation. 1. Clinical notes toward a reconsideration of "adolescent turmoil." *Adolescent Psychiatry, 25,* 3–16.

Eder, D. & Kinney, D. A. (1995). The effect of middle school extra curricular activities on adolescents' popularity and peer status. *Youth & Society, 26,* 298–324.

Edwards, J. (2013). Users on this site have successfully driven nine teenagers to kill themselves. Read more: http://www.businessin sider.com/askfm-and-teen-suicides-2013-9#ixzz2f994TuSF

Elkind, D. (1967). Egocentrism in adolescence. *Child Development, 38,* 1025–1034.

Elkind, D. & Bowen, R. (1979). Imaginary audience behavior in children and adolescents. *Developmental Psychology*, *15*, 38–44.

Fisher, R. M. S. (1991). Pubescence: a psychoanalytic study of one girl's experience of puberty. *Psychoanalytic Inquiry*, *11*, 457–479.

Fonagy, P. (2008). A genuinely developmental theory of sexual enjoyment. *Journal of the American Psychoanalytic Association*, *56*, 11–36.

Freud, A. (1949/1968). On certain difficulties in the preadolescent's relation to his parents. *The writings of Anna Freud*, *4*, 95–106.

Freud, A. (1958). Adolescence. *Psychoanalytic Study of the Child*, *13*, 255–278.

Freud, S. (1919). Lines of advance in psychoanalytic therapy. In J. Strachey (Ed. and Trans.), *The Standard Edition of the Complete Psychological Work of Sigmund Freud* (Vol. 27, pp. 157–168). London: Hogarth Press.

Friedman, R. C. (2001). Psychoanalysis and human sexuality. *Journal of the American Psychoanalytic Association*, *49*, 1115–1132.

Furman, W. & Buhrmester, D. (1992) Age and sex differences in perceptions of networks of personal relationship. *Child Development*, *63*, 103–115.

Galatzer-Levy, R. & Cohler, B. J. (2002). Making a gay identity: coming out, social context and psychodynamics. *The Annual of Psychoanalysis*, *30*, 255–286.

Garcia-Ruiz, M., Rodrigo, M. J., Hernandez-Cabrera, A., Maiquez, M. L., & Dekovic, M. (2013). Resolution of parent-child conflicts in the adolescence. *European Journal of Psychology of Education*, *28*, 173–188.

Garner, R., Bootcheck, J., Lorr, M., & Rauch, K. (2006). The adolescent society revisited: cultures, crowds, climates and status structures in seven secondary schools. *Journal of Youth and Adolescence*, *35*, 1023–1035.

Gilmore, K. (2002). Diagnosis, dynamics, and development: considerations in the psychoanalytic assessment of children with AD/HD. *Psychoanalytic Inquiry*, *22*, 72–390.

Grumbach, H. H. (2002). The neuroendocrinology of human puberty revisited. *Hormone Research in Pediatrics*, *57*(s), 2–14.

Hauser, S. T. & Smith, H. F. (1991). The development and experience of affect in adolescence. *Journal of the American Psychoanalytic Association*, *39S*, 131–165.

Hendry, L. B. & Kloep, M. (2011). A systemic approach to the transitions to adulthood. In, J. J. Arnett, M. Kloep, L. B. Hendry, &

J. L. Tanner (Eds.), *Debating Emerging Adulthood: Stage or Process?* (pp. 53–76.1). Oxford, UK: Oxford University Press.

Jacobs, T. J. (2000). Early adolescence and its consequences. *Journal of Infant, Child & Adolescent Psychotherapy, 1,* 135–157.

Jacobson, E. (1961). Adolescent moods and the remodeling of psychic structures in adolescence. *Psychoanalytic Study of the Child, 16,* 164–183.

Jessor, R. (1977). *Problem Behavior and Psychosocial Development: A Longitudinal Study of Youth.* New York: Academic Press.

Jessor, R. (1991). Risk behavior in adolescence: a psychosocial framework for understanding and action. *Journal of Adolescent Health, 12,* 597–605.

Kaltiala-Heino, R., Kosunen, E., & Rimpela, M. (2003). Pubertal timing, sexual behavior and self-reported depression in middle adolescence. *Journal of Adolescence, 26,* 531–545.

Kernberg, O. F. (2006). Identity: recent findings and clinical implications. *Psychoanalytic Quarterly, 75,* 969–1003.

Knight, R. (2005). The processes of attachment and autonomy in latency. *Psychoanalytic Study of the Child, 60,* 178–210.

Knight, R. (2011). Fragmentation, fluidity, and transformation: nonlinear development in middle childhood. *Psychoanalytic Study of the Child, 65,* 19–47.

Koepke, S., & Denissen, J. J. A. (2012). Dynamics of identity development and separation-individuation in parent-child relationships during adolescence and emerging adulthood—a conceptual integration. *Developmental Review, 32,* 67–88.

Kuhn, D. (2008). Formal operations from a twenty-first century perspective. *Human Development, 51,* 48–55.

Laufer, M. (1976). The central masturbation fantasy, the final sexual organization, and adolescence. *Psychoanalytic Study of the Child, 31,* 297–316.

Laufer, M. & Laufer, E. (1984). *Adolescence and Developmental Breakdown.* New Haven, CT: Yale University.

Laursen, B., Bukowski, W. M., Nurmi, J., Marion, D., Salmela-Aro, K., & Kiuru, N. (2010). Opposites detract: middle school peer group antipathies. *Journal of Experimental Child Psychology, 106,* 240–256.

Laursen, B., Coy, K. C., & Collins, W. A. (1998). Reconsidering changes in parent-child conflict across adolescence: a meta-analysis. *Child Development, 69,* 817–832.

Levy-Warren, M. H. (2008). Wherefore the Oedipus complex in adolescence? Its relevance, evolution, and appearance in adolescence. *Studies in Gender & Sexuality, 9,* 328–348.

Loewald, H. (1979). The waning of the Oedipus complex. *Journal of the American Psychoanalytic Association, 27,* 751–775

Loewald, H. (1985). Oedipus complex and development of self. *Psychoanalytic Quarterly, 54,* 435–443.

Lyons-Ruth, K. (1991). Rapprochement or approchement: Mahler's theory reconsidered from the vantage point of recent research on early attachment relationships. *Psychoanalytic Psychology, 8,* 1–23.

Marohn, R. C. (1999). A re-examination of Peter Blos' concept of prolonged adolescence. *Adolescent Psychiatry, 23,* 3–19.

McHale, S. M., Shanahan, L., Updegraff, K. A., Crouter, A. C., & Booth, A. (2004). Developmental and individual differences in girls' sex-typed activities in middle childhood and adolescence. *Child Development, 75,* 1575–1593.

Mead, M. (1928/2001). *Coming of Age in Samoa: A Psychological Study of Primitive Youth for Western Civilization.* New York: William Morrow & Company.

Mendle, J., & Ferrero, J. (2012). Detrimental psychological outcomes associated with pubertal timing in adolescent boys. *Developmental Review, 32,* 39–68.

Mendle, J., Harden, K. P., Brooks-Gunn, J., & Graber, J. A. (2010). Development's tortoise and hare: pubertal timing, pubertal tempo, and depressive symptoms in boys and girls. *Developmental Psychology, 5,* 1341–1353.

Mendle, J., Turkheimer, E., & Emery, R. E. (2007). Detrimental psychological outcomes associated with early pubertal timing in adolescent girls. *Developmental Review, 27,* 151–171.

Molloy, L., Ram, N., & Gest, S. D. (2011). The storm and stress (or calm) of early adolescent self-concepts: within and between subject variability. *Developmental Psychology, 47,* 1589–1607.

Offer, D. (1965) Normal adolescents: interview strategy and selected results. *Archives of General Psychiatry, 17,* 285–289.

Offer, D. & Offer, J. L. (1968). Profiles of normal adolescent girls. *Archives of General Psychiatry, 19,* 513–522.

Paikoff, R. L. & Brooks-Gunn, J. (1991). Do parent-child relationships change during puberty? *Psychological Bulletin, 110,* 47–66.

Paus, T., Keshaven, M., & Giedd, J. N. (2008). Perspectives: why do many psychiatric disorders emerge during adolescence? *Nature Reviews: Neuroscience, 9*, 947–957.

Peskin, J. & Wells-Jopling, R. (2012). Fostering symbolic interpretation during adolescence. *Journal of Applied Developmental Psychology, 33*, 13–23.

Person, E. (1999). *The Sexual Century.* New Haven: Yale University.

Phinney, V. G., Jensen, L. C., Olsen, J. A., & Cundick, B. (1990). The relationship between early development and psychosexual behavior in adolescent females. *Adolescence, 25*, 321–332.

Piaget, J. (1972). Intellectual evolution of adolescence to adulthood. *Human Development, 15*, 1–12.

Redd, N. A. (2007). *Body Drama.* New York: Gotham Books.

Rosenblum, L. A. (1990). A comparative primate perspective on adolescence. In J. Bancroft, & J. M. Reinisch (Eds.), *Adolescence and Puberty* (pp. 63–69). New York: Oxford University Press.

Rutter, M., Graham, P., Chadwick, O. F. D., & Yule, W. (1976). Adolescent turmoil: fact or fiction? *Journal of Child Psychology and Psychiatry, 17*, 35–56.

Schlegel, A. & Barry, H. (1991). *Adolescence: An Anthropological Inquiry.* New York: Free Press.

Shapiro, T. (2008). Masturbation, sexuality, and adaptation: normalization in adolescence. *Journal of the American Psychoanalytic Association, 56*, 123–146.

Spear, L. P. (2000). The adolescent brain and age-related behavioral manifestations. *Neuroscience & Biobehavioral Reviews, 24*, 417–463.

Spear, L. P. (2004). Adolescent brain development and animal models. *Annals of the New York Academy of Sciences, 1021*, 23–26.

Spear, L. P. (2010). *The Behavioral Neuroscience of Adolescence.* New York: W. W. Norton.

Sroufe, L. A., Bennett, H. C., Englund, M., Urban, J., & Shulman, S. (1993). The significance of gender boundaries in preadolescence: contemporary correlates and antecedents of boundary violation and maintenance. *Child Development, 64*, 455–466.

Steinberg, L. (2000). The family at adolescence: transition and transformation. *Journal of Adolescent Health, 27*, 170–178.

Steinberg, L. (2004). Risk taking in adolescent: what changes and why? *Annals of the New York Academy of Science, 102*, 51–58.

Steinberg, L. (2008). A social neuroscience perspective on adolescent risk-taking. *Development Review, 28,* 78–108.

Stone, L. J. & Church, J. (1955). *Childhood and Adolescence.* New York: Random House.

Sullivan, H. S. (1953). *The Interpersonal Theory of Psychiatry.* New York: W. W. Norton.

Turkel, A. R. (2007). Sugar and spice and puppy dogs' tails: the psychodynamics of bullying. *Journal of the American Academy of Psychoanalysis, 35,* 243–258.

Van Grove, J. (2013). Facebook fesses up: young teenagers are getting bored. http://www.cnet.com/news/facebook-fesses-up-young-teens-are-getting-bored/, October 30, 2013.

Vandenbosch, L. & Eggermont, S. (2012). Understanding sexual objectification: a comprehensive approach toward media exposure and girls' internalization of beauty ideals, self-objectification, and body surveillance. *Journal of Communication, 62,* 869–887.

Wei, C. & Gregory, J. W. (2009). Physiology of normal growth. *Pediatrics and Child Health, 19,* 236–240.

Westen, D. (1990). The relations among narcissism, egocentrism, self-concept, and self-esteem: experimental, clinical, and theoretical considerations. *Psychoanalysis & Contemporary Thought, 13,* 83–239.

Wills, T. A., Resko, J. A., Ainette, M. G., & Mendoza, D. (2004). Smoking onset in adolescence: a person-centered analysis with time varying predictors. *Health Psychology, 23,* 158–167.

Wolf, E., Gedo, J. E., & Terman, D. M. (1972). On the adolescent process as a transformation of the self. *Journal of Youth & Adolescence, 1,* 257–272.

Worthman, C. (1999). Evolutionary perspectives on the onset of puberty. In W. Travathan, E. O. Smith, & J. J. McKenna (Eds.), *Evolutionary Medicine and Health* (pp. 135–163). New York: Oxford University.

7

Middle and Late Adolescence: Sex and Gender, Individuation, and Identity in Progression toward the Threshold of Adulthood

Overview

Social Context

The importance of social context increases exponentially as the adolescent progresses to high school and college or employment. The adolescent and society interact in a dramatically bidirectional dialectic: *Culture* and *youth culture* (see glossary) shape and transform each other. This is the intermediate space in which cultural objects "allow a two-way osmosis between inner and outer" (Bonaminio, 201, p. 102). Adolescence has always marked a dramatic shift in the locus of control from family to society. Not only do relationships with peers, academic demands, and myriad other experiences offered by school, neighborhoods, social networking sites, teams, and clubs absorb and shape the adolescent, but cultural objects— the zeitgeist, the institutions, and the people in the surround— assume dynamic formative functions in the developing mind of the teenager, more or less displacing the family's centrality. Peers, teachers, coaches, schools, gangs, rock stars, celebrities, Facebook, Twitter, Instagram, ask.fm, the current youth culture—these are the people and things that define the world and set the standard for what is beautiful, desirable, sexy, exciting, entertaining, good, and admirable. This change in focus escalates dramatically in high school and college and is typically compounded by the inevitable gap that stretches between youth culture and the parents' generation.

Despite the repetitive nature of generational conflict, some historical moments produce a more discontinuous and disrupted adolescent-to-adult transition. Severe adolescent discontent and/ or alienation as a social phenomenon is highly responsive to cultural, national and international events shaped by technological innovation, tyranny, war, poverty, social injustice, unemployment, technology, and many other factors. For example, the activist youth of the 1960s and 1970s absorbed the attention of key psychoanalytic adolescent commentators, brought central psychological tasks into high relief, and led to lasting contributions from thinkers like Erikson and Blos. Today's social disjunction has many familiar disparities and some that are entirely new. Like generations of parents before them, the current parent generation is ignorant of contemporary trends, innovations, and technology, but the *millennial generation* (Pew Research Center, 2014) (see glossary) differs in consequential ways: In their parents' view, today's teens demand instant gratification, are screen obsessed, exhibitionistic, irresponsible, immoral, and absorbed in virtual reality. Millennials' goals, work ethic, and values seem alien, their romantic/sexual connections superficial, and their shared morals suspect. Although some of these descriptors are typical of parental views of youth culture, social and psychoanalytic observers concur that there has been a seismic shift in Western postindustrial society and in the way adulthood is currently conceptualized. Traditional pathways to adulthood have crumbled, traditional employment opportunities have disappeared, and new technology drives the economy.

Post-postmodern (alternatively called *pseudomodern* or *metamodern*) society has introduced a new sensibility, with a different experience of reality and time, and a different valuation of information. Today's adolescent is highly skilled in the use of electronic devices and knows the terrain of cyberspace far better than the parent generation. Currently, early adolescents have access to an array of social networks, some monitored and some not, and by mid-adolescence, the wider world of the internet is fully available. Parental controls, if attempted, are easily outwitted by teens seeking unhampered access to the site of their choice: Anonymous interactive sites, pornography, paramilitary propaganda sites, instructions for suicide methods, gaming, and gambling sites—indeed, the full gamut of information and exchange available. Moreover, adolescents are the prime target of mass media in its multiple forms and thereby are simultaneously the receivers and creators of societal change as their preferences and trends are carefully monitored and manipulated. Adolescent character formation is clearly affected by the postmodern condition. The ascendance of relativism, the associated unmasking of the word (especially the written word) as coercive, moralizing, and falsely "objective" (Gergen, 1994) the temptations of conventionality (Kernberg, 1989), the acculturation to visual media, self-transformation, and gratification through virtual reality (Lemma, 2010), and the pervasive post-postmodern skepticism (Eizirik, 1997) are only beginning to be felt as today's emerging adults attempt to grow up and assume leadership.

Mid-adolescence

Of all the subphases in the adolescent process, the mid-adolescent period is perhaps the most peer-obsessed, media-drenched, and present-oriented (Levy-Warren, 1996). A drive to act in the real world, take risks, seek new sensations, and explore the hitherto barred adult activities reflects a confluence of developing systems. The individuation process requires aggressive defiance of parental codes and restrictions, and the search for identity presses the adolescent into active collision with the world (Chused, 1990). The ongoing asynchrony among impulses, judgment, and self-regulation fuels escalating risky behaviors despite demonstrable evidence of improving judgment (Steinberg, 2004) and capacity to reflect (Westen, 1990).

Teens entering high school have passed through the peak velocity of their physical development and have usually achieved relative stabilization of adolescent hormonal fluctuations. Their sense of themselves as gendered and sexual is established, although confusion about orientation and subjective gender definition may persist, and their actual sexual experience is usually limited. High school, anticipated with excitement and dread as a legendary cauldron of breathtaking adventures, illicit substances, and sexual exploits, is now an imminent reality. The mid-adolescent faces the challenge of negotiating this social minefield without the reassurance or constraints of parental approval and guidance. The power of the internalized representation of the parental voice continues to wane and the mid-adolescent must go it alone. This evolution is exacerbated by the inevitable parent generation's "ignorance" of youthful trends and desires, now more pronounced by the shift to a technology-driven culture. The struggle for distance from parents and their internalized voices, however actively sought, contributes to a sense of alienation and existential loneliness, even while surrounded by peers (Berman, 1970; Blos, 1967). Adolescent alienation from the adult world at large is the cultural extension of this process; its severity ebbs and flows from generation to generation in relation to current social issues, specific youth culture, and political climate (Arnett, 2004; Wise, 1970).

In general, the intrapsychic representations of primary objects undergo considerable transformation through the early phase of individuation, optimally permitting *object removal* (Katan, 1951) (see glossary); that is, the successful shift of libidinal focus away from parents to the peer group, without the requirement of an actual rupture (Besser & Blatt, 2007). Nonetheless, conflict with parents is a common feature in this cohort. Its positive correlation with success in establishing romantic relationships (Dowdy & Kliewer, 1998) suggests that the "removal" of romantic and sexual feelings to the peer group both reinforces and is reinforced by the assertion of autonomy from parents. The superego of latency, based on internalization of parental injunctions, is weakened and/ or re-externalized onto authority figures over the course of adolescence, and the mid-adolescent increasingly turns to the peer group for guidance and standards. The rate of conflict with parents may decline from early adolescence, but the affect intensity of such conflicts peaks during high school years (Laursen et al., 1998). Sexual experience and romance are an overriding focus for the mid-adolescent. Noncoital "hooking up" (a sexual encounter without expectation of a relationship) begins in late middle school or early high school; by the end of mid-adolescence (roughly age 17–18), the majority of teens will have their first experience of intercourse (Pederson, Samuelson, & Wichstrom, 2003). As noted, self-paced sexual encounters are opportunities for self-discovery as a sexual and embodied person and actually contribute to well-being, if in keeping with group norms. Although reports vary, it appears that sexual activity in pace with the peer group is generally experienced as positive by both girls and boys: The teens lagging behind are the ones who suffer in terms of confidence and self-esteem (Vrangalova & Savin-Williams, 2011). Moreover, despite contemporary depiction of "hook ups" as pervasive, impersonal, and indiscriminate, closer examination shows that in this age group they are typically between individuals who are familiar and repeat partners. Often, at least one of the two involved hopes that these encounters will eventually lead to a relationship (Manning, Giordano, & Longmore, 2006). However, the subjective experience of hook-ups changes with age, becoming far less satisfying for late adolescents.

Electronic media is increasingly prominent and absorbing to adolescents. Teens spend roughly one-third of each day on the internet (Escobar-Chavez & Anderson, 2008), which offers access to a host of sites, from pragmatic to entertaining, where they can get school reading lists and assignments, plan social events, explore pornography, play games, including massively multiplayer online role-playing games (MMORPGs), research topics both academic and otherwise, and learn about the college process (Wohn et al., 2013) in addition to engaging in destructive pursuits such as stalking, cyber-bullying, internet gambling, researching weapons and suicide methodology, and obsessiveness about any of these. Mid-adolescents rely on daily access to messaging apps and social networking sites such as ask. fm, Instagram, and Tumblr as their twenty-first century version of the suburban mall. Gossip, displays of popularity, and voyeuristic

"stalking" of love interests or rivals are routine fare. In more problematic applications, cyberspace offers adolescents struggling with
the reality of their transformed and sexualized bodies a virtual
universe in which the actual corporeal self is left behind and the
self-representation is reinvented at will (Lemma, 2010).

As noted, the normative identity crisis is a process that today
extends over almost two decades. Kernberg (2006) called it the most
visible manifestation of the individuation process. As adolescents
extricate themselves from the network of "identifiers" developed
over childhood that defined and positioned them in their family
culture, they encounter a different series of limiting environments
and subcultures. Adolescent identity development, beginning with
the momentous entry into middle school, is under continuous construction but remains subject to environmental feedback. Because
the transition from middle to high school can range from seamless
to transformative, both within the individual and in the immediate environment, the opportunities to explore and discover new
facets to identity are similarly variable. Even with the transient
decline in academic performance, related to a predictable uptick in
academic challenge and complexity (Isakson & Jarvis, 1999), entry
into high school is often personally liberating; it offers access to a
larger, more diverse peer group and greater choice of extracurricular
activities, with potential for self-discovery and relationship development based on shared interests. Moreover, because up to 90% of
American high school youth between sophomore and senior year
have had some form of employment outside the academic sphere,
pre-career employment provides auxiliary role experimentation, in
addition to fostering work ethic, personal agency, and autonomy.
This impressive statistic may be driven by the loss of vocational
training in high school curricula. High schoolers who are steadily
employed over long periods of time under low intensity conditions
(<20 hours per week) are more likely to attend and graduate from
college (Zimmer-Gemback & Mortimer, 2006).

There is consensus that with age, social dominance structures
decline. Middle school is described as a harsher world than high
school; the stereotypic consensual categorizations acquired there

(usually "popular and unpopular") eventually yield to more personal and nuanced assessments of other people frequently reported by students toward the end of their final year of high school. Adolescent society is clearly embedded in and shaped by environmental factors. The degree to which academic performance, admission to college, and athletic excellence are endorsed in the community certainly affects the nature of high school groups (Garner, Bootcheck, & Michael, 2006). High school cliques formed around interests, sports, academics, and other extracurriculars, ultimately decline as teens expand horizons. In communities in which college is the goal of high school, grades, extracurriculars, and the more judicious use of social media in the junior and senior year are powerfully influenced by the wish to impress college admissions committees.

Late Adolescence

As with all phases of adolescence, the timing and focus of late adolescence is a complex product of today's culture and timeless aspects of mental life. Although mid-twentieth century scholars viewed the college experience as a problematic overextension of the adolescent process (Blos, 1967; Erikson, 1956), most came to agree that the 18 to 23 year old was appropriately still grappling with adolescent tasks (Adatto, 1991; Blos, 1962, 1967; Erikson, 1956; Ritvo, 1971), at least in the Western culture under observation. The psychological tasks of late adolescence are a continuation of central adolescent challenges, specifically individuation, identity exploration, further reintegration and modification of the superego, and intimate romantic relationships. This phase is supported by the foundation established during the earlier adolescent phases, including the integration of the sexual body and physical development, and growing consciousness of a future in the "real world."

Today, the majority of American youth[1] enter college following high school. Contemporary cultural factors powerfully shape the late adolescent experience by the following means: (1) High school guidance has undergone ideological shift toward promoting higher education in order to fulfill the presidential "college for all" mandate (Rosenbaum, 2011), preparing young people for an increasingly challenging job market. Despite persistent differences in the opportunities and developmental trajectories of teenagers based on socioeconomic status, high schoolers are now routinely funneled into college prep and deflected from vocational training. (2) A college degree has become mandatory for decent job opportunities—it is the "new" high school diploma.[2] (3) The institutional authority of colleges has declined with the explicit rejection of *in loco parentis* beginning in the 1960s (Whitaker, 2011). (4) Adult markers (independent financial status and domicile, marriage, childbearing, established career) are significantly delayed relative to 50 years ago (Arnett, 2000).

Today's impressive college entry statistic does not speak to the rate of graduation,[3] but it does demonstrate that the majority of post–high school youth get a taste of the institutional *psychosocial moratorium* (Erikson, 1956, 1965) (see glossary), wherein the important tasks of late adolescence can be addressed in a permissive context, subsidized, as it were, by parents or other resources (Ritvo, 1971). Despite the contemporary reality that entry into college does not ensure clarification of career goals or even a degree within six years, any time spent on campus widens horizons previously limited by family, neighborhood, and high school culture. The psychosocial moratorium facilitates developmental tasks, including the *second individuation* (see glossary), identity integration, intimate relationships, the setting of personal values and ideals, and the sense of responsibility for oneself and ones choices. For contemporary late adolescents, the accomplishment of these tasks herald the attainment of adulthood. Indeed, "the two top [self-selected] criteria for the transition to adulthood in a variety of studies have been accepting responsibility for one's self and making independent decisions" (Arnett, 2000, p. 473). The simple reality that college usually entails geographical separation from family, however wrenching, is often salutary in and of itself. In general, the college experience allows new opportunities to elaborate, repair, or rewrite identity; new perspectives on family culture and values; new degrees of freedom from supervision; infinite choice of mentors, activities and focus; self-governance and the possibility of experimentation in a range of arenas. The college student is mandated to discover passions, rework values and moral beliefs, and determine what matters. At the same time, none of these mandates are consequential. There is freedom from full financial responsibility; exploration can take many turns before approaching commitment. It is a dress rehearsal or intermediate step toward independence, on a smaller stage than the "real life" that remains in the distance until graduation approaches.

Late adolescents are capable of more self-reflection and consciousness of their own narratives, past and future. The deepening of cognitive capacities associated with perspective-taking and abstract thinking makes the average late adolescent "less of a demographer, less of a behaviorist, more of a psychological clinician. Expressed in broadest terms, with increasing age the child becomes less of a Skinnerian, more of a Freudian" (Rosenberg, 1979, p. 202). This cognitive maturity also promotes the evolution of identity as a mental construct, refines the identity-related self-representation, integrates the information about one's identity reflected in the eyes of others, and consolidates the cohesive narrative arc of the autobiographical self with a past and a future.

Undoubtedly college also has the potential to impose its own stereotyping and limit the promise of infinite horizons by institutional tendencies toward monolithic identities. Athletic teams, Greek life (fraternities and sororities), sober dorms, math majors lend themselves not only to caricature but also to discrepant internal representations that compete for "temporal and psychological resources" (Killeya-Jones, 2005). Racial, gender-related, religious, and ethnic attributes, in addition to interests and talents, can force individuals into roles defined by consensual expectations; because identity is always in context, it evolves in dialectic exchange with subculture (Eichler, 2011; Steele, 1997). College life is also replete with invitations to engage in risky behaviors that are augmented by the (relative) absence of restrictions, access to illicit substances, sexual freedom, and minimal oversight of college personnel. Such opportunities, seized indiscriminately by previously sheltered teens, can yield identity labels such as "sexually promiscuous," "party animal," and so on, which adhere despite efforts to change.

In spelling out late adolescent tasks, psychoanalytic thinkers of the mid-twentieth century recognized that adolescent "closure" and consolidation of the adult personality organization are processes not necessarily completed even during college. These observers, writing in the 1950s and 1960s, documented sustained internal struggle in adolescents and young adults despite the fact that the manifest indications of adulthood were achieved earlier then than they are today.[4] The notion that "establishment of a mature personal, ethnocultural, spiritual and sexual identity" (Kline, 2006) is fully completed in late adolescence is incompatible with the reality that identity is a continuous process in interaction with the environment (Lewis & Mayes, 2012). On the level of life decision making, the experience of today's 18 to 23 year old is rarely informed by the idea that the future must be finalized by age 25; delays in making definitive choices, for example in regard to career and life partner, defines this cohort. The extended time frame for adolescent resolution in contemporary Western society highlights the fact that the "psychological and reality tasks of adulthood" (Ritvo, 1971) can remain unaddressed and unfinished into the late twenties.

Teenagers who enter the workforce immediately after high school are in the minority in the current "college-for-all" climate. This group is identified as socioeconomically disadvantaged, urban, poor, learning disabled, and/or minority students who have not been prepared to meet the academic demands of college; in fact, they are handicapped from early childhood when expectations about college are observed to begin. By the time they enter high school, these children's intentions to *not* pursue undergraduate education are solidly established (Grodsky & Riegle-Crumb, 2010), and only a confluence of exceptional personal capacities and fortuitous events can create a different orientation: for example, their "discovery" by families or teachers as possessing academic or artistic potential or their own inspiration by an encouraging role model. Opportunities for role exploration, mentoring, and "semi-autonomy" decline in the full-time workforce; in contrast, these are amply available to the college student (Zarrett & Eccles, 2006, p. 19). The likelihood of heading directly from high school to a career-oriented and growth-promoting job—especially one that facilitates independent living, promises personal development, and offers a vision of the future—is unfortunately not improved by prior part-time employment, because the latter usually bears little relationship to ultimate career direction (Zimmer-Gemback & Mortimer, 2006). For most late adolescents going directly into the work force, the decade following high school is typically spent in a series of jobs (on average seven) that only stabilizes as these youth approach 30 (Hamilton & Hamilton, 2006). This pattern may be likened the role exploration permitted in college, but it is more consequential when conducted in the working world and entered into the "permanent record" of work history.

The full-time late adolescent worker is likely to be relatively unsupervised, unless the young person has the good fortune to obtain unofficial guidance and support. Only the military offers a setting comparable to college or the vocational training of past generations. In the armed forces, skill training and competence development are explicit agendas, the step away from the home environment is concretely supported by provision of room and board, and the demand for discipline compensates for loss of parental guidance and ensures focus and cooperation.

Studies of "hook-up culture"—that is, a culture in which traditional dating is eclipsed by casual sexual encounters (typically occurring at parties and usually with a known hook-up partner) with no expectation of commitment—demonstrate that although the term "hooking up" has been used since the 1980s, its dominance seems to be a more recent phenomenon. The percentage of students who have hooked up at least once increases over the course of high school; in college, where this culture has been most observed and studied, the number follows a steep upward ascent, and the experience has increasing negative valence for both males and females. A recent review of the existing literature found that two thirds to three fourths of college students hook up at least once in college, and one in five have hooked up 10 or more times

(Heldman & Wade, 2010). Various societal trends are cited as contributions: increased access to pornography, co-ed dorms, a rise in alcohol use on campuses, a "pornification" of media representations of men and women, a decline in the perception of risk in regard to sexually transmitted diseases (Heldman & Wade, 2010), and a cultural devaluation of deep intimate relationships in favor of "autistic autosensuousness" (Bonaminio, 2014, p. 100).

Individuation

As described in the introduction to adolescence, Blos's conceptualization of the second individuation (1967) as a central task of adolescence, based on Mahler's separation–individuation paradigm, has had detractors over its history, especially as it was grounded in classical psychosexual developmental theory and was interpreted as normalizing a break away from parents driven by incestuous anxiety (Marohn, 1999). As noted, an inevitable violent rupture is not supported by empirical research (Offer, 1965), but discernible stirrings of individuation are documented in pre- and early adolescence by the mounting intergenerational tension. By mid-adolescence parent–child conflict declines in frequency but is marked by more heated and hostile emotions (Laursen et al., 1998). The content of conflict increasingly concerns the teen's privacy and autonomy, regardless of varying family culture and ethnicity: "I'm not trying to disrespect them, just make my own life" (Phinney et al., 2005, p. 31); "get out of my life, but first could you drive me and Cheryl to the mall?" (Wolf, 1991); "I just gotta have my own space" (James, 2001) are a sampling of mid-adolescents' sentiments, informed by the determination to redefine themselves and palpably less focused on parents as arbiters or judges.[5]

Anticipation of college in the immediate future can rekindle old conflicts and anxieties. Because emancipation from the rule of internalized infantile objects is a gradual process that evolves throughout adolescence, it may founder as the college-bound teen contemplates the concrete geographical remove and associated loss of parental guidance, supervision, and constraints. Anxiety in anticipation of separation from the family is often obscured by absorption in the events before departure: the college process itself, with its associated competition, expectations, disappointments, and excitement; the imposed shifts in identity as applicants receive the "verdict" from their college choices and this in turn is inevitably made public; the new discoveries, interest in, and bonding with their high school cohort; the realization of the imminent loss of familiar peer relationships.

For those high school juniors and seniors whose autonomy and individuation have depended on the reassuring push-back of parents/teachers/boarding school resident assistants (i.e., trained peer advisors assigned to a residence hall) and the like—whether as supports or containers for externalized superego injunctions—preparations for college may elicit surprising regressive or oppositional tendencies. Adequate prior management of age-related separations (for camp, class overnight trips, and the like) does not guarantee success in the remarkably unstructured and non-authoritarian setting of college. In fact, establishment of intrapsychic autonomy in mid-adolescence rather than a history of uneventful separations, is a prognostic indicator for success in the early years of college life. Adjustment depends on the "balance between object closeness and object distance in relationships with significant others" that reflects progression in the intrapsychic process of individuation (Holmbeck & Wandrei, 1993, p. 75). Incoming college freshman who have not progressed sufficiently in establishing this balance become symptomatic early in their college careers. These are the students who are swept up in risky behaviors without apparent capacity to self-monitor, who appear depressed and unmotivated to attend classes, or who urgently seek a replacement for the parental presence such as a new love relationship or excessive dedication to a fraternity or sorority. Such individuals may decline rapidly, unable to establish appropriate functional independence and reliable internal self-regulation. They soon manifest disorganization, regressive behavior, and need to return home. Despite the correlation of problematic family environments with poor initial adaptation to colleges

(Holmbeck & Wandrei, 1993), these late adolescents often benefit from a semester or full academic year at home, augmented by short "internship" programs that promote agency, independent decision making, and responsibility. Psychological treatment at this juncture is likely to be brief for pragmatic reasons, but can help to establish enhanced individuation, differentiated management of conflict, and disengagement from a problematic role or foreclosed identity fostered by the family of origin. Even short-term interventions may allow these students to return to college better individuated and more able to rely on internal sources of stability and guidance.

Blos (1954) described a more pathological variant of adolescent process, which he called *prolonged adolescence* (see glossary). He limited his description to boys, but included features that are observable in many college students who struggle with the challenges of the late adolescent process. In his cohort, the problem begins with excessive prepubertal narcissism fostered by an overidealization of the boy by his mother. Entering the new world of college with its unprecedented challenges, he is unable to tolerate exposure and to risk the effort necessary to fulfill her expectations. There is minimal intrapsychic conflict and no internal pressure to conclude the adolescent process. These are students who maintain expectations of greatness without willingness to compete and to strive for the less glorious achievements of good grades.

The pathologic suspension of time in this syndrome highlights the transformation of time sense during adolescence that Seton calls adolescent "psychotemporal adaptation" (Seton, 1974). No doubt *technoculture* (see glossary) is transforming this process in the twenty-first century, because the usual constraints imposed by the clock are abolished in virtual reality. Instant gratification, access to content well beyond developmental level or psychic comprehension, such as pornography and violent videos, and exposure to media that promotes early sexualization are just a few of the time-bending features of cyberspace. Seton suggests that the growing awareness of one's separate history, ordered by time and memory into a narrative life story with a past, present, and future, is an integrative achievement of late adolescence. It reflects the successful negotiation of individuation and active identity formation. The orientation of today's emerging adults is demonstrably not toward a settled future when examined in the context of ongoing risk behaviors (see chapter 8); how post-college recklessness influences late adolescents' capacities to look forward has yet to be determined.

The Identity Crisis

Erikson's status as a psychoanalytic thinker and theoretician has been compared with Freud's in the "socio-historical surround of world culture" (Wallerstein, 1998, p. 230). His contributions to conceptualization of the life span and specifically to late adolescent development have generated a vast body of research (operationalized as *identity status* (see glossary); see Marcia, 1966), and theoretical literature (Kroger, 2004). The description of the identity crisis in adolescence and the problem of its resolution have been fundamental to the study of late adolescence and the passage to adulthood, and are central to theories of personality disorders (Kernberg, 2006). But despite broad influence on developmental science and related fields, Erikson's theory has, historically, been marginalized in the psychoanalytic community as "sociological" (E. Jacobson, quoted in Wallerstein, 1998, p. 231), because it focuses on the interface of psyche and society. It has received scant psychoanalytic endorsement and minimal efforts to coordinate it with psychoanalytic developmental literature. In our view, Erikson's emphasis—on the complex, multifaceted interaction of intrapsychic processes of personality consolidation and self-representation, as these are both shaped and reflected back by environmental response—is unavoidable, because it is the heart of the adolescent process. Identity achievement, like adulthood itself, is shaped by cultural opportunity, realized through social institutions, and validated by significant others. The intrapsychic events of this period are deeply embedded in and affected by the surround (Blum, 2010).[6]

Erikson's concept of a normative developmental crisis specific to adolescence is not meant to restrict the process of identity formation even to the whole sweep of adolescence and emerging adulthood. Throughout his writings, he reiterates that identity begins with childhood identifications and evolves through middle childhood. With adolescence, these identifications undergo a process of transformation, selection, and repudiation—consciously, preconsciously, and unconsciously—to establish a "new configuration" that is recognized by the environment (1956, p. 68) and gradually stabilizes to reflect "both a persistent sameness within oneself [self-sameness] and a persistent sharing of some kind of essential character with others" (Erikson, 1956, p. 57).

Thus, identity is an extraordinarily complex and encompassing aspect of personality—an amalgam of conscious and unconscious elements with a long intrapsychic evolution—meriting its designation as a developmental line. Many of the conscious components are more or less immutable, often passed down from generation to generation or bestowed at birth, like race, sex, cultural, ethnic and/ or religious heritage, or place in birth order. Other components are mostly unconscious: identifications with parents promoting mental structure, especially superego formation; identifications forged out of the need to differentiate from siblings (Vivona, 2007); and identity elements accrued in relation to subjective experience of gender and sexuality, interaction with the social world, and other *component identities* (see glossary). Each of these conscious and unconscious, longstanding or recent components—including gender identity, sexual orientation identity, relationship identity, career identity, ethnic identity, religious identity, political identity, and so on—has its own history within individual development and ebbs and flows in its prominence in self-representation and personal narrative, depending on developmental level and context. In addition these components bear on the question of moral compass, beliefs, and values and so interface with superego evolution. As identity consolidates over the course of adolescence, many of these elements are radically reworked, revised or reconsidered.

The various domains of identity require reciprocal "acknowledgment of these role commitments and self-views by the broader community" (Wilkinson-Ryan & Westen, 2000, p. 529). These domains, although not entirely independent, do not develop in lockstep. Their achievement implies synthetic capacity, self-regulation, self-coherence, and internal representations that guide behavior (Bradley & Westen, 2005, p. 936). Identity is a construct that overlaps with the concept of the self as elaborated by self-psychologists (Wallerstein, 1998). It requires progress toward individuation as described by Blos, and implies reintegration of superego values, which in the ideal case appear fully operational in and inseparable from personality. Although not emphasized in Erikson's work, identity is powerfully linked to adolescent bodily transformation, egocentrism, and emerging formal operations: introspection, heightened awareness of one's inner life and other's perceptions, and the growing depth of interpersonal experience all figure in the process of identity formation (Rosenberg, 1979; Westen, 1990).

When the search for identity becomes a conscious focus, what Erikson calls extreme "identity consciousness" (1956, p. 74), experimentation does not lead to resolution in a timely fashion and every move forward is fraught with the awareness of being watched. Erikson emphasizes that the identity process fluctuates;intervals of confusion are inevitable, even desirable, and do not indicate psychopathology provided there is continued movement. This is borne out by "identity status" research findings that document the gradual progression from confusion toward achievement (or foreclosure) over the college years (Kumru & Thomson, 2003; Meeus et al., 1999). Erikson observed that advances toward identity achievement impart a subjective experience of "psychosocial well-being ... a feeling of being at home in one's body," a sense of "knowing where one is going," and "an inner assuredness of anticipated recognition from those who count" (Erikson, 1956, p. 74).[7] This echoes Blos's view that adolescent character formation creates a sense of being "at home." Indeed, the developmental processes of ego integration, individuation, self-formation,[8] and personality consolidation, emphasized by other psychoanalytic thinkers, are in large part compatible with Erikson's thinking and seem to operate in pace with identity formation.

The entire sdolescent period involves reworking childhood identifications and new component aspects. Late adolescence (18–22) has been documented in the research literature to be the most active period for identity formation (Kumru & Thomson, 2003). Of course, ultimate identity achievement is necessarily a composite structure that is more than the sum of its parts. Ongoing striving for autonomy and individuation works synergistically with this integrative process. The college experience can serve as a facilitator through provision of the psychosocial moratorium in which the normative identity crisis occurs in a protected, sanctioned environment. Many late adolescents use this new setting to break free of the social hierarchies of high school, the constraints of prior self-representations as endorsed and fostered by peers and family, and the confines of family microculture in relation to sexuality, religion, ambitions, and many other arenas. They make use of exposure to the diversity and opportunities provided by college life and time abroad. These environments facilitate the synthetic process of identity formation, which integrates past childhood editions and evolving new identifications (Erikson, 1956). However, as we discuss in chapter 8, identity achievement recently accomplished in the college setting may not carry forward into the "real world." The latter poses a new set of challenges not necessarily anticipated in the college setting.

Intimate Relationships

As noted, contemporary hook-up culture is a lesser factor in mid-adolescence and tends to cluster with other risk behaviors (Fortunato et al., 2010). However, hook-up culture dominates the college scene with problematic impact on late adolescents. In the aftermath of hooking up, it appears that regret and reputation damage are gender specific along conventional lines: Girls suffer more than boys (Heldman & Wade, 2010; McHugh, M. Pearlson, & Poet, 2012). Moreover, the hook-up dominated social scene does not foster sustained love affairs, and the important developmental experience of intimate relationships is short-circuited (Barber, 2006). Casual and meaningless sexual encounters do little to weave together the triad of lust, romantic love, and attachment that mediate intimacy and contribute to the powerful state alterations associated with the early stages of falling in love (Fisher, 2006; Yovell, 2008). But it is also true that this triad forms a complex system with mutual influence (i.e., lust can influence attachment, attachment can produce love, and so); many casual relationships, so-called "friends with benefits," have all the elements present, but weighted differently. At least some of those "playing the game" get hooked on each other (Schwartz, 2006) and proceed into long-term relationships.

Certainly romantic, sexually intimate peer relationships are still valued as peak emotional experiences and potential sources of deep gratification and well-being. For the late adolescent, the experience of falling in love requires that the autonomy and sense of self so recently achieved gives way to the relaxation of hard-won boundaries in order to depend on another person both emotionally and physically (Kernberg, 1974; Ritvo, 1971) and to allow the melding of oedipal love and idealization of the primary objects of infancy into the intoxicating state of love (Solnit, 1982). Progress toward the establishment of autonomous identity is usually foundational for romantic love (Beyers & Seiffge-Krenke, 2010), but passionate love relationships themselves can foster and enhance identity features that rest on narcissistic and moral capacities. Romantic, erotic, committed love relationships bring together strands of tenderness, desire, idealization, trust, faithfulness, and the capacity to rely on another while elevating self-esteem and confidence. Falling in love requires sufficient superego stability to accommodate "hitherto forbidden wishes, as well as feeling states" (Ross, 1991, p. 471), and to sustain fidelity (if agreed upon) against temptation. In Kernberg's view, the capacity for romantic relationships is a complex accomplishment:

> The achievement of this stage of development of internalized object relations brings about the transformation of body surface erotism into tenderness, of need-gratifying relationships into object constancy, and, together with the capacity for mourning,

guilt, and concern, results in a deepening awareness of the self and of others, the beginning of the capacity for empathy and for higher level identifications. (1974, p. 748)

This description highlights ego capacities that emerge and evolve through adolescence, including deepening tolerance for both sublime and painful affects, self-reflection and "thinking about thinking," acceptance of responsibility, the ability to see the perspectives of others, and a willingness to aspire to ideals. Such developments evolve in direct relationship to superego maturation.

Superego

Over the course of mid- to late adolescence, the superego undergoes multiple transformations, progressing from the relatively comfortable late latency incarnation to the early to mid-adolescent expulsion, and finally to late adolescent reintegration, now shaped by individuated ideals, goals, and moral values. The re-externalization of childhood injunctions and the reliance on the peer group for standards and ideals in mid-adolescence are driven by burgeoning sexuality, incestuous anxiety, the need for object removal, and early attempts to individuate by opposition and alienation from shared familial beliefs. As the sexual self becomes integrated into identity, individuation becomes more secure, and the ego's deployment of defenses stabilizes, a dialogue with primary objects becomes possible. However reluctantly, the late adolescent not only recognizes and tolerates parents' flaws—their sexual lives and moral failings—but also sees their positive qualities. Despite this détente, adolescents in high school and college more often turn to others—self-selected mentors among their teachers, coaches, political heroes, or intellectual titans—who embody newly embraced values and accomplishments. These contribute to the adolescent reworking of the superego to represent fully individuated standards and aspirations.

The term *ego ideal* is used inconsistently in psychoanalytic literature. In Blos' theorizing (1972), the ego ideal emerges in tandem with the matured superego at the termination of late adolescence, bringing together components of infantile grandiosity and the subsequent childhood idealization of the same-sex parent: The ego ideal is the "heir of the negative oedipal complex" (Blos, 1972, p. 96). In optimal developmental circumstances, the adolescent process will transform these precursors into "a firm guide to action" and "... the guardian of the sense of integrity, self-esteem, and love of the self" (p. 97). This latter description approximates the use of the term by other authors as the repository of abstracted moral standards, independent of specific admired individuals ("idols") or narcissistic self- aggrandizement (Laufer, 1964; Milrod, 1990, 2002). This definition of the ego ideal distinguishes it from narcissistic strivings from its inception: It is a metaphorical yardstick of moral purity and goodness, a substructure of the superego. In contrast, the "wished-for-self-image" (Milrod, 1990) is an ego structure based on strivings for coveted attributes that can be traced to preoedipal yearnings for narcissistic gratifications like (super) power and adoration. Morality is never entirely clean of self-interested motivations, but the distinction between the ego ideal and the narcissistically driven "wished-for-self-image" highlights an important distinction between, on the one hand, standards of moral goodness and the guilt associated with failure to achieve them and, on the other, fantasies of wealth, power, beauty, thinness, muscularity, or other coveted attributes whose lack elicits shame. The ego ideal fosters late adolescents' pursuit of "noble purpose" (Bronk, 2011), epitomized by service activities following college such as the Peace Corps or "Teach for America," whereas the wish-for-self-image promotes the self-interested dedication to making lots of money, achieving celebrity, and gaining power.

There are indications that contemporary western techocultural society may be inadvertently supporting sustained splitting of drive components and sequestering action from superego oversight. Impulses that gradually come under aegis of superego prohibition and/or ego regulation are instead exercised at will in the free-for-all, anonymous virtual world. By providing a "hidden" outlet for flagrant, unbridled perverse and aggressive activities, cyberspace becomes a dangerous playground for the mid- and late adolescent. The typical offenses of the internet—cyber-bullying, stalking, hacking, and perverse sexual behaviors—are often committed by young people whose moral values and actual behavior appear well-regulated. Moreover, the overt activities of social media typically demand the sacrifice of personal privacy in exchange for the excitement of exhibiting and looking, with potential hypertrophy of these drive derivatives. How misuse of the internet figures into late adolescent personality integration is yet to be fully realized or understood.

Onset of Psychiatric Illness

Late adolescence, as defined here, marks the onset of the majority of psychiatric illnesses, including mood disorders and substance abuse. Although the actual onset of schizophrenia is difficult to determine in many cases, it too is considered to begin before age 24 (Kessler et al., 2007). In addition, onset of personality disorders, no longer restricted to those over 18 years of age by DSM criteria, are increasingly diagnosed in mid- to late adolescence. The psychoanalytic conceptualization of the process of personality consolidation in the final phase of the adolescence, now stretched into the twenties, suggests that there may still be potential growth in defenses, superego structure, and ego capacities to rework ominous traits and manage the predilection toward impulsive action. Some prominent psychoanalytic contributors have maintained that personality disorders can be traced to patterns observed in childhood (P. Kernberg et al., 2000), but psychiatric researchers support the more optimistic view that innate resilience, environment, and experience can intervene to create a different outcome (Paris, 2003; Rutter, 1987).

Summary

The period that begins with entry into high school and extends to age 22, 23, or 24 encompasses a remarkable transition in adolescent development. The path from the anxious high school freshman, at the threshold of the exciting and dangerous contemporary youth culture, to the graduating college student or young worker who confronts the sobering reality of adulthood in the contemporary world, is full of developmental opportunity and pitfalls. It follows the arc from fantasy and anticipation through the action-orientation of mid-adolescence, to the late adolescent consciousness of future reverberations of current decisions that must be made with care.

"Coming of age" is not only about becoming a sexually equipped and experiencing person, but also coming into the epoch that defines the generation. The crucial preparation for adulthood includes the twin processes of individuation and identity formation, the consolidation of superego, the resolution of residual childhood trauma, and the settling of gender identity and sexual orientation. "Psychotemporal adaptation" (Seton, 1974) implies that the adolescent experiences him- or herself as a recognizable continuous entity, with a childhood past and, by the end of late adolescence, an eye trained on future actualization. Contemporary technoculture is transforming this process in myriad ways: deleteriously, by unbridled, anonymous opportunities to commit and/or witness acts formerly forbidden, by heightening voyeuristic observation and exhibitionistic displays of inflated, even patently false self-representations, and by the associated corruption of standards. On the positive side, the digital world promotes awareness and tolerance in regard to cultural differences, offers vast new economic opportunities, and sustains relationships over distances readily traversed by today's globalized youth. The impact of cyberspace and technoculture can reverberate, for better or worse, in superego modifications, stabilization of identity, self-representation, and evolving notions of love, sex, and relationships, and thus may ultimately lead to significant generational differences in developmental outcome.

Central points about mid- to late adolescence include the following:

- Mid-adolescence is used here to designate the high school-aged child, roughly 14 to 18. During this phase the child's focus is fixed on the peer group and, gradually, his or her own (immediate) future. This era usually includes stabilization of physical growth, with consolidation of the self-representation as a sexual person. In addition, intimate relationships assume growing significance. Preparation for life after high school graduation and anticipation of geographic separation from home and family occupies the teenager approaching the end of this phase.

- Late adolescence here refers to individuals between 18 and 24, the majority of whom attend college in the United States. College provides the institutional psychosocial moratorium that allows these late adolescents a setting and opportunities to explore and experiment with whom they are and whom they want to be. Whether at school or on the job, identity formation interacts with the individuation process to promote a coherent sense of a separated, directed life. Identity is composed of component elements that can progress unevenly; some are determined at birth, some imposed by society, and some are self-selected. Superego stabilization and growing capacity to engage in intimate sexual relationships are the crowning achievements of these two phases.

Notes

1. Sixty-six percent, according to the 2012 Bureau of Labor Statistics News Release.

2. The New York Times, February 19, 2013: *It takes a B.A. to find a job as a file clerk*, by Catherine Rampell.

3. In 2011, the six-year graduation rate was 58% of enrollees, according to the US Department of Education report: *The Condition of Education 2011*.

4. In 1960, the accomplishment of "adult tasks" (marriage, career choice, child bearing) among 25 year olds was achieved by 68% of

females and 44% of males, whereas today only 25% of females and 13% of males have done so (Furstenberg, 2010).

5. Paradoxically, mid-adolescents' immersion in contemporary technology means they can access the "mall of today" without needing their parents for transportation and that "their own space" (i.e., their room or, more abstractly, their privacy) is actually (virtually) populated by their peer group, envied clique, love interest, or object of stalking.

6. Now that the enterprise of psychoanalysis itself is in danger in a culture that is globalized, deluged with information, used to rapid, if not instant, gratification, and in which hallowed institutions are rapidly disappearing, more psychoanalytic attention is focused on the profound effect of shifting priorities and the interpenetration of our society with character formation during adolescence (Eizirik, 2009; Galatzer-Levy, 2012). Hopefully, both psychoanalysis and the traditional pillars of identity (that is, commitment to roles, self-continuity over time and in a range of circumstances, the sense of inner agency, responsibility, preservation of values, and sense of purpose) will survive.

7. A comprehensive review of this literature showed that identity foreclosure was also associated with well-being (Meeus et al., 1999).

8. Erikson's relative neglect in psychoanalytic literature has been compounded by the lack of official recognition that the rise of self-psychology (Kohut) owes a great deal to Erikson's elaboration of identity as a hybrid mental construct (Wallerstein, 1998).

References

Adatto, C. P. (1966). On the metamorphosis from adolescence into adulthood. *Journal of the American Psychoanalytic Association, 14,* 485–509.

Adatto, C. P. (1991). Late adolescence to early adulthood. In S. Greenspan, & G. Pollock (Eds.), *The Course of Life.* Vol. IV, *Adolescence* (pp. 357–375). Madison, CT: International Universities Press.

Arnett, J. J. (2000). Emerging adulthood: a theory of development from the late teens through the twenties. *American Psychologist, 55,* 469–480.

Arnett, J. J. (2004). *Adolescence and Emerging Adulthood: A Cultural Approach.* Boston: Prentice Hall.

Auchincloss, E. A. & Samberg, E. (2012). *Psychoanalytic Terms & Concepts*. New Haven, CT: Yale University Press.

Barber, B. L. (2006). To have loved and lost…adolescent romantic relationships and rejection. In A. C. Crouter & A. Booth (Eds.), *Romance and Sex in Adolescence and Emerging Adulthood* (pp. 29–40). New York: Psychology Press.

Berman, S. (1970). Alienation: an essential process of the psychology of adolescence. *Journal of the American Academy of Child Psychiatry, 9,* 233–250.

Besser, A. & Blatt, S. J. (2007). Identity consolidation and internalizing and externalizing problem behaviors in early adolescence. *Psychoanalytic Psychology, 24,* 126–149.

Beyers, W. & Seiffge-Krenke, I. (2010). Does identity precede intimacy? Testing Erikson's theory on romantic development in emerging adults of the 21st century. *Journal of Adolescent Research, 25,* 387–416.

Blos, P. (1954). Prolonged adolescence: the formulation of a syndrome and its therapeutic implications. *American Journal of Orthopsychiatry, 24,* 733–742.

Blos, P. (1962). *On Adolescence: A Psychoanalytic Interpretation*. Glencoe, NY: Free Press.

Blos, P. (1967). The second individuation process of adolescence. *Psychoanalytic Study of the Child, 22,* 162–186.

Blos, P. (1972). The function of the ego ideal in adolescence. *Psychoanalytic Study of the Child, 27,* 93–97.

Blos, P. (1979). *The Adolescent Passage: Developmental Issues*. New York: International Universities Press.

Blum, H. P. (2010). Adolescent trauma and the oedipus complex. *Psychoanalytic Inquiry, 30,* 548–556.

Bonaminio, V. (2014). "A perfect world" and its imperfections: psychoanalytic clinical notes on adolescence and virtual reality. In A. Lemma & L. Caparrotta (Eds.), *Psychoanalysis in the Technoculture Era* (pp. 97–113). London: Routledge.

Bradley, R. & Westen, D. (2005). The psychodynamics of borderline personality disorder: a view from developmental psychology. *Development & Psychopathology, 17,* 927–957.

Bronk, K. C. (2011). The role of purpose in life in healthy identity formation: a grounded model. *New Directions in Youth Development, 2011,* 31–44.

Bureau of Labor Statistics, Economic News Release: College Enrollment and Work Activity of 2012 High School Graduates. United States

Department of Labor, April 17, 2013, http://www.bls.gov/news.
release/hsgec.nr0.htm

Chused, J. F. (1990). Neutrality in the analysis of action-prone adolescents. *Journal of the American Psychoanalytic Association, 38,*
679–704.

Dowdy, B. B. & Kliewer, W. (1998). Dating, parent-adolescent conflict,
and behavioral autonomy. *Journal of Youth and Adolescence, 27,*
473–492.

Eichler, R. J. (2011). The university as a (potentially) facilitating environment. *Contemporary Psychoanalysis, 47,* 289–316.

Eizirik, C. L. (1997). Psychoanalysis and culture: some contemporary
challenges. *International Journal of Psychoanalysis, 78,* 789–800.

Escobar-Chavez, S. L. & Anderson, C. (2008). Media and risky behaviors. *Future of Children, 18,* 147–180.

Erikson, E. H. (1956). The problem of ego identity. *Journal of the
American Psychoanalytc Association, 4,* 56–121.

Erikson, E. H. (1965). *Identity: Youth and Crisis.* Austen-Riggs
Monograph Series. New York: W. W. Norton.

Fisher, H. (2006). Broken hearts: the nature and risk of romantic rejection.
In A. C. Crouter & A. Booth (Eds.), *Romance and Sex in Adolescence
and Emerging Adulthood* (pp. 3–29). New York: Psychology Press.

Fortunato, L., Young, A. M., Boyd, C. J., & Fons, C. E. (2010). Hook-up
sexual experiences and problem behaviors among adolescents.
Journal of Child & Adolescent Substance Abuse, 19, 261–278.

Furstenberg, F. F. (2010). On a new schedule: transitions to adulthood
and family change. *The Future of Children, 20,* 67–87.

Galatzer-Levy, R. (2012). Obscuring desire: a special pattern of male
adolescent masturbation, internet pornography, and the flight
from meaning. *Psychoanalytic Inquiry, 32,* 480–495.

Garner, R., Bootcheck, J., & Michael, L. R. (2006). The adolescent society revisited: cultures, crowds, climates, and status structures in
seven secondary schools. *Journal of Youth and Adolescence, 35*(6),
1023–1035.

Gergan, K. J. (1994). Exploring the postmodern: perils or potentials?
American Psychologist, 49, 412–416.

Grodsky, E. & Riegle-Crumb, C. (2010). Social background and college
orientation. *The Annals of the American Academy of Political and
Social Science, 627,* 14–35.

Hamilton, S. F. & Hamilton, M. A. (2006). School, work and emerging
adulthood. In J. J. Arnett & J. L. Tanner (Eds.), *Emerging Adults*

in America: Coming of Age in the 21st Century (pp. 257–277). Washington, DC: American Psychological Association.

Heldman, C. & Wade, L. (2010). Hook-up culture: setting a new research agenda. *Sexuality Research & Social Policy, 7*, 323–333.

Holmbeck, G. N. & Wandrei, M. L. (1993). Individual and relational predictors of adjustment in first-year college students. *Journal of Counseling Psychology, 40*, 73–78

Isakson, K. & Jarvis, P. (1999). The adjustment of adolescents during the transition into high school: a short–term longitudinal study. *Journal of Youth and Adolescence, 28*, 1–26.

James, K. (2001). "I just gotta have my own space!": the bedroom as a leisure site for adolescent girls. *Journal of Leisure Research, 33*, 71–90.

Katan, A. (1951). The role of "displacement" in agoraphobia. *International Journal of Psychoanalysis, 32*, 41–50.

Kernberg, O. (1974). Mature love: prerequisites and characteristics. *Journal of the American Psychoanalytic Association, 22*, 743–768.

Kernberg, O. (1989). The temptations of conventionality. *International Journal of Psychoanalysis, 16*, 191–205.

Kernberg, O. (2006). Identity: recent findings and clinical implications. *Psychoanalytic Quarterly, 75*, 969–1003.

Kessler, R. C., Amminger, G. P., Aguilar-Gaxiola, S., Alonso, J., Lee, S., & Ustan, B. D. (2007). Age of onset of mental disorders: a review of recent literature. *Current Opinions in Psychiatry, 20*, 359–364.

Killeya-Jones, L. A. (2005). Identity structure, role discrepancy and psychological adjustment in male college student. *Journal of Sport Behavior, 28*, 167–185.

Kline, R. B. (2006). *Principles and Practices of Structural Equation Modeling* (2nd ed.). New York: Guilford Press.

Kumru, A. & Thompson, R. A. (2003). Ego identity status and self-monitoring behavior in adolescents. *Journal of Adolescent Research, 18*, 481–495.

Kroger, J. (2004). *Identity in Adolescence: The Balance between Self and Other* (3rd ed.). Hove, UK: Routledge.

Laufer, M. (1964). Ego ideal and pseudo ego ideal in adolescence. *Psychoanalytic Study of the Child, 19*, 196–221

Laursen, B., Coy, K. C., & Collins, W. A. (1998). Reconsidering changes in parent-child conflict across adolescence: a meta-analysis. *Child Development, 69*, 817–832.

Lemma, A. (2010). An order of pure decision: growing up in a virtual world and the adolescent's experience of being-in-a-body. *Journal of the American Psychoanalytic Association, 58,* 691–714.

Levy-Warren, M. (1996). *The Adolescent Journey: Development, Identity Formation, and Psychotherapy.* New York: Jason Aronson.

Lewis, M. & Mayes, L. C. (2012). The role of environment in development: an introduction. In L. C. Mayes & M. Lewis (Eds.), *The Cambridge Handbook of Environment in Human Development* (pp. 1–12). Cambridge, UK: Cambridge University Press.

Manning, W. D., Giordano, P. C., & Longmore, M. A. (2006). Hooking up: the relationship contexts of "nonrelationship" sex. *Journal of Adolescent Research, 21,* 459–483.

Marcia, J. E. (1966). Development and validation of identity status. *Journal of Personality and Social Psychology, 3,* 551–558.

Marohn, R. C. (1999). A reexamination of Peter Blos's concept of prolonged adolescence. *Adolescent Psychiatry, 23/24,* 3–19.

McHugh, M. C., Pearlson, B., & Poet, A. (2012). Who needs to understand hook-up culture? *Sex Roles, 67,* 363–365.

Meeus, W., Ledema, J., Helsen, M., & Vollebergh, W. (1999). Patterns of adolescent identity development: review of the literature and longitudinal analysis. *Developmental Review, 19,* 419–461.

Milrod, D. (1990). The ego ideal. *Psychoanalytic Study of the Child, 45,* 43–60.

Milrod, D. (2002). The superego: its formation, structure, and functioning. *Psychoanalytic Study of the Child, 57,* 131–148.

Offer, D. (1965). Normal adolescents; interview strategy and selected results. *Archives of General Psychiatry, 17,* 285–289.

Paris, J. (2003). *Personality Disorders over Time: Precursors, Course, and Outcome.* Washington, DC: American Psychiatric Press.

Pederson, W., Samuelson, S. O., & Wichstrom, L. (2003). Intercourse debut age: poor resources problem behavior, or romantic appeal? A population based longitudinal study. *Journal of Sexual Research, 4,* 333–345.

Pew Research Center. (2014). Millennials: a portrait of generation next. http://pewresearch.org/millennials/

Phinney, J. S., Kim-Jo, T., Osorio, S., & Vilhjalmsdotir, P. (2005). Autonomy and relatedness in adolescent-parent disagreements: ethnic and developmental factors. *Journal of Adolescent Research, 20,* 8–39.

Ritvo, S. (1971). Late adolescence—developmental and clinical considerations. *Psychoanalytic Study of the Child, 26*, 241–263.

Rosenbaum, J. (2011). The complexities of college for all: beyond the fairy-tale dreams. *Social Education, 84*, 113–117.

Rosenberg, M. (1979). *Conceiving the Self.* New York: Basic Books.

Ross, J. M. (1991). A psychoanalytic essay on romantic, erotic love. *Journal of the American Psychoanalytic Association, 39S*, 439–475.

Rutter, M. (1987). Psychosocial resilience and protective mechanisms. *American Journal of Orthopsychiatry, 57*, 316–331.

Schwartz, P. (2006). What elicits romance, passion, and attachment and how do they affect our lives throughout the life cycle? In A. C. Crouter & A. Booth (Eds.), *Romance and Sex in Adolescence and Emerging Adulthood* (pp. 49–60). New York: Psychology Press.

Seton, P. H. (1974). The psychotemporal adaptation of late adolescence. *Journal of the American Psychoanalytic Association, 22*, 795–819.

Solnit, A. J. (1982). Developmental perspectives on self and object constancy. *Psychoanalytic Study of the Child, 37*, 201–218.

Steele, C. (1997). A threat in the air: how stereotypes shape intellectual identity and performance. *American Psychologist, 52*, 613–629.

Steinberg, L. (2004). Risk taking in adolescence: what changes and why? *Annals of the New York Academy of Science, 102*, 51–58.

Vivona, J. M. (2007). Sibling differentiation, identity development, and the lateral dimension of psychic life. *Journal of the American Psychoanalytic Association, 55*, 1191–1215.

Westen, D. (1990). The relations among narcissism, egocentrism, self-concept, and self-esteem: experimental, clinical, and theoretical considerations. *Psychoanalysis and Contemporary Thought, 13*, 183–239.

Vrangalova, Z. & Savin-Williams, R. C. (2011). Adolescent sexuality and positive well-being: a group-norms approach. *Journal of Youth and Adolescence, 40*, 931–944.

Wallerstein, R. S. (1998). Erikson's concept of ego identity reconsidered. *Journal of the American Psychoanalytic Association, 46*, 229–247.

Whitaker, L. C. (2011). College student psychotherapy in cultural and institutional context. *Contemporary Psychoanalysis, 47*, 317–328.

Wilkinson-Ryan, T. & Westen, D. (2000). Identity disturbance in borderline personality disorder: an empirical investigation. *American Journal of Psychiatry, 157*, 528–541.

Wise, L. J. (1970). Alienation of present-day adolescents. *Journal of the American Academy of Child Psychiatry, 9*, 264–277.

Wohn, D. Y., Ellison, N. B., Laeeq Kahn, M., Fenwins-Bliss, R., & Gray, R. (2013). The role of social media in shaping first-generation high school students' college aspirations: a social capital lens. *Computers & Education, 63,* 424–436.

Wolf, A. E. (1991). *Get out of My Life, but First Could You Drive Me and Cheryl to the Mall?* New York: Noonday Press.

Yovell, Y. (2008). Is there a drive to love? *Neuropsychoanalysis, 10,* 117–144.

Zarrett, N. & Eccles, J. (2006). The passage to adulthood: challenges of late adolescence. *New Directions for Youth Development, 111,* I13–28.

Zimmer-Gemback, M. J. & Mortimer, J. T. (2006). Adolescent work, vocational development, and education. *Review of Educational Research, 76,* 537–566.

8

Emerging Adulthood and Contemporary Society: Development in the Third Decade

Overview

A Problem of Definition

Adult development has long been a controversial topic in the psychoanalytic literature. This chapter addresses the contemporary interest, originating within the allied fields of developmental psychology and sociology, in the proposal of a new developmental phase, *emerging adulthood*: youth who stand between adolescence and adulthood, neither teenagers nor grown-ups. An immediate definitional problem confronts the reader of both the psychoanalytic and development literature about this topic, because, as noted in our introduction to adolescence, subphases and the boundaries of young adulthood are demarcated inconsistently and differ not only in the popular press, but also from one researcher or thinker to another in consequential ways. Moreover, given the disillusionment with the notion of developmental phases altogether, it seems all the more remarkable that a new one has been proposed (Arnett et al., 2011; Hendry & Kloep, 2007).

What and When Is Emerging Adulthood?

As noted in chapter 6, G. Stanley Hall's tour de force introduction to adolescence at the turn of the twentieth century (1904) identified a phase of development that, with the exception of pubertal events, had received little scholarly attention. Hall argued that the adolescent process spanned the decade between 14 and 24, extending from the then-contemporary median age of menarche to the typical age of adult commitments (marriage, career, and childrearing). Even with lower rates of college attendance at the turn of the century, limiting the opportunity for identity exploration, Hall maintained that adolescence continued into the mid-twenties. His description alerted scientists and researchers to a multifaceted era of bio/psycho/social development that had gone unstudied and now became the subject of vast scientific and literary interest. Adolescence is firmly established as a legitimate developmental epoch, with a new mental organization, a set of daunting tasks and challenges, remarkable changes in brain and body, and the emergence of a complex set of new capacities in emotions, thinking, self-representation, relationships, sexuality, and so on.

In the context of the growing college attendance by American children in the second half of the twentieth century, sociologists and psychoanalytic thinkers grappled with the timing of the adolescent phenomenon: Some viewed the college experience as an unnatural extension of the process, but gradually most concurred that adolescence does not end at age 18. These observers placed late adolescence and the segue to adulthood in slightly different time frames and gave the transition different names: "youth" (Keniston, 1968), "postadolescence" (Blos, 1962), or the "psychosocial moratorium" (Erikson, 1956). The question of whether this period constitutes a separate subphase of adolescence or represents early adulthood was not a focus, in part because these adolescent specialists all considered social factors to play a key role in the transition. Jeffrey Arnett, who coined the term *emerging adulthood* (2000) for people between the ages of 18 and 24 or 25, renewed widespread interest in the adolescent to adult transition.[1] Arnett finds support for his proposal in the work of the mid-century adolescent scholars, Erikson (1956) and Blos (1954), who initially responded to the marked uptick in college attendance with the concern that the adolescent to adult transition had been stretched out, perhaps excessively. Arnett's time frame corresponds with the final years of adolescence in Hall's thinking, resembles aspects of Blos' description of pathological *prolonged adolescence* (see glossary) or normal "postadolescence," and incorporates Erikson's idea of the psychosocial moratorium (see glossary) provided by the college experience. Arnett's depiction of the "state" of emerging adulthood s closely resembles Erikson's description of the period of psychosocial moratorium that facilitates the establishment of identity:

> Emerging adulthood is distinguished by relative independence from social roles and from normative expectations. Having left the dependency of childhood and adolescence, and having not yet entered the enduring responsibilities that are normative in adulthood, emerging adults often explore a variety of possible life directions in love, work, and world-views. Emerging adulthood is a time of life when many different directions remain possible, when little about the future has been decided for certain, when the scope of independent exploration of life's possibilities is greater for most people than it will be at any other period of the life course. (Arnett, 2000, p. 469)

Arnett's five criteria are identity-centric and difficult to distinguish from what we have included in the core challenges of late adolescence (Arnett, 2004, p. 8):

1. Identity explorations
2. Instability
3. Heightened self-focus
4. Subjective feeling of being in-between
5. Age of possibilities

In our sequence, the four to five years after high school graduation (the years of college or early employment in a "McJob" [Coupland, 1991]) are late adolescence proper; the future and adulthood are acknowledged but safely shelved. The years that follow, up until the late twenties, more typically include a conscious and unconscious transition into adulthood that is strongly shaped by environmental conditions in contemporary society. Whether or not there is associated ongoing psychological transformation and development sufficient to merit a new phase, the existence of the *millennial odyssey* (Brooks, 2007) (see glossary) is undeniable and has been amply documented in the scientific and lay press Indeed, despite our disagreement with his time frame, we believe that Arnett has pointed out a real generational phenomenon, illuminating the plight of the 23- or 24- to 30-year-old in contemporary society (Arnett, 2007).

Arnett readily admits that emerging adulthood is the outcome of societal changes that have visibly influenced and expanded the developmental process. To the extent that adolescence is "an act of man" invented to describe the transition from childhood to adulthood (Blos, 1979), emerging adulthood is yet another man-made construction—the contemporary extension that further prolongs the transition. The multiple transformations in turn-of-the-twenty-first century Western society have resulted in delays in the achievement of the typical markers of adulthood. Traditionally, these markers included the conventions of maturity, such as establishing a personal domicile apart from parents, entering a career path, committing to marriage, and planning for childrearing (Bynner, 2005). Of course, these measurements of adulthood rely on elective choices deeply shaped, paced, and emphasized or de-emphasized by the culture in which they occur. Moreover, they reflect the reality that as adulthood approaches, the biological driver wanes in importance, making way for the augmented shaping role of social trends and opportunities. It remains to be seen whether the expectation of an extended odyssey (Brooks, 2007) toward adult status through the twenties affects the maturation of cognition, personality synthesis, and consolidation of adult *identity components* (see glossary). Alternatively, it may reflect changes in prior developmental periods that impede the approach to adulthood.

Does this phase, regardless of time frame, require Arnett's new terminology? Detractors in sociology and developmental psychology object to emerging adulthood as another example of simplistic phase thinking; reifying it as a phase belies its transitory existence as an epiphenomenon of social change and obscures the huge variability among individuals in their twenties (Bynner, 2005; Hendry & Kloep, 2007). However convincing their argument for its impermanence may be, their socioeconomic perspective may not give sufficient weight to the impact of the computerized, globalized, cyberspatial world on psychic development. Other commentators see the post-postmodern and *technoculture era* (see glossary) as effecting profound transformations in the mental organizations of young people. These, in turn, may result in irreversible transformations in representations of adulthood and its goals, with repercussions extending into earlier development.

Simply on the level of its pragmatic value, we endorse the use of omnipresent phase terminology. Because social forces invariably partner with biological maturation to drive and shape development, the delineation of phases highlights the powerful interface between cultural institutions and mental life, nowhere more apparent than in regard to adolescence and adulthood. Arnett's formulation draws attention to the contemporary reality that today's late adolescents, in college or workforce, are not striving to conclusively achieve the hallmarks of adulthood. They enter their mid-twenties "milling about" (Tanner, 2006, p. 43) with a sense of suspension that is disconcerting to both them and their parents. Those who attended college, even if successfully graduated, are uncertain about their future trajectory and return to the parental home without a job or meaningful career path. Those whose education ended with high school (typically low income, and racially, culturally, and linguistically diverse) also demonstrate lack of focus: Stabilization and lengthening stints in jobs only occur as age 30 approaches (Hamilton & Hamilton, 2006). Committed intimate adult relationships are further delayed; moreover, marriage is no longer a subjective badge of adulthood. Although these traditionally defined adult markers—marriage or career path—do still occur, they occur significantly later than half a century ago (Arnett, 2005; Furstenberg, 2010). To the degree that they play a role in ego consolidation, in addition to reflecting its progress, the synergy is dissipated.

As noted, today's prolongation of adolescent closure has been widely recognized in developmental literature and the popular press. Coincidentally, new findings from contemporary neuroscience document brain changes through the third decade of life (Lebel & Beaulieu, 2011)Association fibers proliferate and shift in function throughout adolescence and young adulthood (Lebel & Beaulieu, 2011) in the wake of the massive synaptic pruning that begins in early adolescence. Although not conclusively linked to behavioral and cognitive manifestations, these neuroanatomic changes suggest that emerging adulthood may indeed have a biological driver. The evidence for a truly novel mental organization is less promising, even though cognitive maturation and deepening expertise clearly occur. At this point in time, emerging adulthood, as defined by Arnett, can be understood as a continuation of the mental organization and the neuroanatomic scupting of late adolescence stretched into the third decade rather than a quantum shift. Although its prolongation has significance for mental life, it is not a new organization, notwithstanding the potential reassurance that the idea of "brain changes" offers to emerging adults and their parents as a physiologic rationale for "wandering" and uncertainty (Beck, 2012). Nonetheless, Arnett's formulation, future neuroscientific advances, and the growing body of research on this population may eventually unveil intrinsic transformations of the mind and brain, not only in the content and connections, but also in the structuralization of the superego,[2] the stabilization of customary defenses and adaptations, the emergence of new ego capacities, and the development of new levels of mentalization and expertise (Blakemore, 2012). It might then qualify, just as adolescence did a century earlier, as a developmnental phase by more stringent criteria. If, in addition, more profound intrapsychic changes are observed, in regard to conceptualizations of reality, time, and meaning, then transformations in multiple systems may be underway. Of note is the observation that the findings about the odyssey years have already had a significant impact on the preceding phase. Late adolescents experience considerably less social pressure to "decide" anything and the consolidation of personality is arguably slowed.

The Particular Challenges of Today's Young Adults

A number of social factors unique to the twenty-first century have contributed to the scholarly interest in this age group at this moment in Western (particularly North American) culture: (1) The "college for all" policy has decreased the cohort of high school students anticipating entry into the work force by seeking appropriate vocational training. (2) The same policy is likely responsible for the significant increase in the percentage of adolescents who enter college compared with a half century earlier.[3] College offers the experience of broad socialization, epitomized by a liberal arts education and the emphasis on training young men and women to think for themselves, but it does not typically funnel them into specific vocational preparation for the future (Arnett & Taber, 1994). (3) As noted, the remarkable college attendance statistic is not matched by similar graduation results.[4] (4) A significant number of both college grads and/or dropouts enter into the workforce without demonstrable expertise or direction. A college diploma confers an advantage only in the hiring process.

Moreover, the turn to a postindustrial, technology-based economy has been accompanied by the decline of traditional pathways to employment. As this generation enters the workforce, it faces unchartered territory. Recession continues to contract the job market, hallowed institutions and career paths are crumbling, parents have little experience negotiating the world of technology in order to advise their adult children, who, as noted, are frequently ill-prepared educationally to enter the job market and achieve financial independence. Past generations of youth who received vocational training or entered preprofessional tracks in college had this relatively unsung advantage. They could turn to parents and other adults as mentors and models. Their schooling provided preparation for future employment. Given the pace of technologic advances and the rapid transformation of proven routes to careers, today's twenty-somethings, the vanguard generation of the digital revolution, are at a disadvantage in terms of their educational preparation; they did not learn code in preschool (see Hu, 2013). Their parents have relatively little first-hand experience to guide their sons and daughters into an alien world (Beyers & Seiffge-Krenke, 2010; Konstam, 2007). The lack of visible pathways to adult roles and the change in the valuation of adult responsibilities may interfere with the intrapsychic stabilization of patterns of adaptation and defense and the process of identity formation. Thus, the extension of the transitional period between late adolescence and adulthood into the twenties can be understood as the outward manifestation of a particular generation grappling with adulthood in dynamic interaction with a transforming world.

Moreover, as the norms for the achievement of the markers of adulthood now drift into the late twenties and their status as accomplishments decline, a period of confusion and wandering seems inevitable: many young people are unprepared to grapple with wide-open career choices, feel confused about paths to success in the void created by their parents' unfamiliarity with contemporary road maps, experience both relief and regression as they return to the parental home, or at the very least are financially dependent on parents.[5] Those with college degrees face the job market with some advantage over their less educated peers, but without having figured out "what to be." The tension between the developmental task of commitment to an adult self-representation and the contemporary environmental deficit in terms of models, opportunities, institutions, guidelines, and even appreciation, produces generations mired in the process of "emerging" all through their twenties.

Contemporary social forces are thus clearly at play in extending late adolescent entry into adulthood. As the time between college and the assumption of adult roles and responsibilities stretches, it seems inevitable that the subjective experience of this age group is affected (Arnett, 1997). The loosened parental constraints, availability of parental financial support, absence of normative shifts inducting the adolescent into traditionally defined adulthood (Hendry & Kloep, 2002), and overall delayed societal expectations to assume the "chains" of adulthood (Colarusso, 1991, p. 127) have a number of psychological corollaries. The inner drive toward autonomous living is diminished. "Feeling young" and with reduced expectations to be "grown-up" makes the time in the twenties "a gratifying ally of the impulses" (Colarusso, 1991, p. 127). The breakdown in traditional models and values alters the desirability of adult status. Today's twenty-somethings, relieved of pressure and ambition to achieve adulthood, are likely to continue the risky behaviors of their early teen years; for example, alcohol consumption peaks at age 26 (Arnett, 2005) and risk behavior in general increases from college levels (Eitle, Taylor, & Eitle, 2010). Planning for adult commitments and the psychological "recentering" (Tanner, 2006) of responsibility associated with that planning appear to be dubious goals. As a consequence, current twenty-somethings may feel distinctly invalidated by adults whose expectations (for settling down, marriage, children, and career path) are premature and/or misguided, if not hypocritical, in contemporary society and who do not see or appreciate other signs of personality consolidation.

Psychoanalytic Contributions

As noted, a number of psychoanalytic observers remarked on a major transformation occurring toward the end of the adolescent process, bridging late adolescence to young adulthood. Although formulations differ, these psychoanalytic clinicians seemed to be addressing the same critical transition, one that could certainly extend into the late twenties and look like Arnett's emerging adulthood. Their proposals share a recognition that a "developmental" intrapsychic process is underway, resulting in the transformation of childhood adaptations and partial solutions into the structured adult character or the adult neurosis (Blos, 1972). These contributors are not proposing new capacities or mental structure, but rather a new integration, new content, and new balance in the agencies of the mind.

Psychoanalytic thinkers in this group describe the process in slightly different ways. Blum (1985) calls it "the final transformation of the personality," including significant revisions of the superego and consolidation of identity. Adatto (1966) describes it as an "intrapsychic metamorphosis" marked by "narcissism in the service of the ego" (p. 502); that is, self-love and self-focus in order to do the work of reintegration of the personality. The strengthening of the ego shifts the ego–superego balance, so that the superego can be modulated to permit full development of sexuality, the establishment of self-determined values and ideologies, and the striving toward personal fulfillment. The somewhat chaotic mobility of mental structure in adolescence ideally resolves into an adaptive, flexible personality. In Adatto's view, the process of psychic reorganization makes the adolescent temporarily intolerant of the regression and the disorganization that is required for analytic work.

Blos (1968, 1972) elaborated the tasks of adolescence that must be managed in order to "resolve" the adolescent process and form the adult character. These include the second individuation, the integration of childhood trauma, the stabilization of sexual identity (referring to sexual orientation and gender identity), and the establishment of ego continuity. Their resolution requires the work of ego consolidation, a manifestation of the synthetic function that weaves patterns of ego attitudes stabilized by identifications (the character traits of childhood) into the stable character of adulthood. In this process, traits are ideally "emancipated from infantile bondage," no longer serve defensive purposes and become flexible "ego assets" via sublimation (1968, p. 248). Character functions as a homeostatic structure integrating ego identifications, defensive patterns, self-esteem, self-concept, and reactions to external stimuli, thereby establishing a reliable set of internal invariants: "one's character is one's home . . . a protector of the self" (Blos, 1968, p. 260). This is the achievement of postadolescence (Blos, 1962; Tanner, 2006).

Many of these conceptualizations arose from observing the transition to adulthood on college campuses in the 1960s and 1970s and from the clinical challenge of working with troubled late adolescents (Adatto, 1966; Blos, 1972; Laufer, 1978). Disagreements about how to intervene with the latter highlight the importance of this developmental process for adult personality organization. To Laufer, intervention is essential to prevent stabilization of pathological intrapsychic solutions, specifically for the adolescent conflict around the sexual body. It is therefore a crucial moment for analytical treatment (Laufer, 1978). However, to Adatto (1966) and Blos (1972), late adolescents do not generally produce a workable transference neurosis for an extended period during the opening phase of analytic work. The final developmental process resists the necessary return to infantile positions and impedes transference crystallization, creating a "stimulus barrier" against the potentially overwhelming recreation of childhood states in the analytical relationship. According to Blos, interpretive work is best limited to fostering awareness of mental life and psychic determinism, whereas the intrapsychic process of analyzable structuralization occurs silently outside the treatment relationship. To Colarusso (1991) and Adatto, "the massive reorganization of the psychic apparatus" (Adatto, 1966, p. 486) effected by this process is fundamentally resistant to analytic work. Blos contends that consolidation can be waited out or even hastened in a preparatory phase of treatment, provided it can be sustained without transference interpretation. To him, childhood conflict and maladaptive solutions do not prevent the advent of the final adult organization, and the latter is more accessible to analysis if achieved in an ongoing therapeutic relationship.

Putting aside the treatment debate, it is clear that these clinicians conceptualize the completion of adolescence as an active intrapsychic process, one that is affected by environmental impingements as well as internal reorganization. The transformation is not evenly achieved across domains (Hendry & Kloep, 2007) or from one moment to the next (Adatto, 1966) and remains susceptible to attenuation or delay imposed or mediated by contemporary societal forces such as the ones described in regard to today's youth and society at large. Like all developmental accomplishments, especially in the adolescent and young adult, these are in constant interaction and transaction with individual psychology and the environment. The systems in transformation include the achievement of full sexual maturity, stabilization of preferred forms of arousal, gender representations, and sexual orientation; resolution of identity in a range of arenas—relational, vocational, aspirational; and consistency in the deployment of patterned defenses, sublimations, and modes of gratification. These achievements blend into processes different from developmental ones, such as stable compromise formations that sustain both neurotic and adaptive patterns, maturation, specialization, and expertise.

New Issues for Identity Achievement

As today's late adolescent college students progress into the twenties, many feel an imminent loss of identity. They approach commencement ceremonies with growing uncertainty and without confidence that they can see a clear path to adulthood. The challenge of identity consolidation can be undermined by the realization that the identity successfully embraced as a college student is not readily transferable to the world at large, neither in terms of content or the value it confers. Reasons for such limitations are varied: the tight embrace of a previously endorsed identity as conferred by family, social status, wealth, and so on may have bypassed exploration, especially if it functions well on campus. Similarly, the reflexive assumption of a "negative" identity—the opposite of what one's parents (or one's college) stand for—offers quick closure to the exploratory process without providing future direction in the world outside. These are known as "foreclosed" identities in the research literature on *identity status* (Marcia, 1993) (see glossary). Active participation in a sport, extracurricular activity such as theater, or a sorority can result in powerful allegiances, values, and self-definition. Success and celebrity on campus derived from these memberships not infrequently fail to offer useful pathways to future roles and gratifications. Whether or not these ultimately endure as important components of self-representation, they may falter or lead to missteps in the harsh outside world. The college football star is not guaranteed a place on a professional team or the social fame, notoriety, and/or power enjoyed at school. All these processes of identity achievement, which may appear as solutions in college, can thus evaporate without the support of the group or the required refitting to measure up to the demands of "real life."

This is perhaps the subtext of David Foster Wallace's commencement address: *This Is Water*.[6] College is a moratorium, true, but it is yet another not-fully-realized particular type of water that young people are swimming in. The identity that has felt so self-selected and directed now confronts life after college. This is not an easy transition, equivalent to culture shock. In its more pathological variant, a college niche can be recruited unconsciously as a bulwark against genuine identity consolidation and autonomy. In such cases, a psychic dead end awaits the graduated young adult stripped of its provision of support, importance, and purpose (Fabricius, 1998).

Occupational identity is clearly an important conscious component of identity consolidation; as aspiration, it more or less guides late adolescent choices of major, study abroad, extracurriculars, internships, grant applications, and the like. The quest for "what to be" reflects the search for an occupation that will eventually provide a livelihood, but more importantly, one that confers (or promises to confer) an identity that both taps aptitudes and interests and connects to the idealized objects of childhood. Moreover, the quest is for naught if the young person does not find a setting in which it is recognized. Such a task requires considerable inner psychological work: discovering one's capacities; managing expectations derived from the wished-for self-image and realistic self-assessment, as well the expectations of others; coming to understand what matters; finding internal resources to realize one's goals. Conscious pressure coming from within—such as the desire to establish financial independence and the quest for a "noble purpose" and meaningful commitment (Bronk, 2011), and from without—such as expectations and standards of family and peers, can rush the time required for this process, leading to a series of missteps. This is especially a problem for today's youth, who often cannot find knowledgeable adults as they consider occupations unfamiliar to the parent generation and observe paths to success that appear to have no real relationship to traditional work ethics, like overnight multimillionaires from start-up IPOs and celebrity ascent from "reality" TV.

Until 1970, Erikson used the terms identity confusion and *identity diffusion* (see glossary) inconsistently in his writings to distinguish between a normative developmental process and a pathological one. In an attempt to clarify his meaning, he noted that adolescents grappling with the identity crisis actually seek a degree of diffusion, namely:

> ... experiences in which some boundaries of the self are sacrificed for a sense of wider identity, with compensatory gains in emotional tonus, cognitive certainty and ideological conviction; all of which occurs in states of love, sexual union, and friendship, of discipleship and followership, and of creative inspiration. (1970, p. 15)

Unfortunately, the term *identity confusion* (which Erikson defines as "an impoverishment and a dissipation of emotional, cognitive, and moral gains in a transitory mob state or in renewed isolation—or both"; 1970, p. 15) has taken on the normative meaning, and identity diffusions used by Kernberg and others has come to designate psychopathology. Erikson's confusion and Kernberg's diffusion are pathological syndromes resembling Blos' prolonged adolescence. These disorders should be distinguished from the extended process of "emerging" currently encountered in young people in their mid-twenties (Wallerstein, 1998). The problematic syndromes, prolonged adolescence and identity diffusion (as defined by Kernberg, 2006), are manifestations of an unresolved identity crisis that persists without closure, resulting in poorly integrated self- and other-representations with little capacity for true intimacy; failure to consolidate of ideals and aspirations; the avoidance of choice; a sense of paralysis and resistance to competition and striving; a disturbance in time sense so that there is simultaneous urgency and lack of impetus, childishness and grandiosity; terror of change together with unrealistic, passive expectations of change through the mere passage of time (Blos, 1954; Kernberg, 2006). Psychopathology is suggested when individuals rely on the adoption of "negative identities" indefinitely, defying expectations of significant others and contradicting their own childhood values. To Erikson, there is an expectable ebb and flow of identity confusion and clarity over the course of adolescence. The prevalent extension of this identity process into the twenties appears to characterize a generation with its own demographics (Arnett, 2000), a particular sociocultural dilemma, and a new set of expectations about consolidating plans. In our experience, along with active exploration and searching, there is mounting anxiety as age 30 approaches.

Shifts in Behavior and Relationships

Emerging adults' relationships with family depend on the mutual recognition that, despite the (hopefully transient) return to the parental home, they have achieved a new level of adulthood and autonomy. The recentering of power and decision making onto the adult child, a process that evolves over late adolescence into the twenties, facilitates improvement in parent–child relations (Tanner, 2006). Relationships with siblings decline in intensity, but if sufficiently relieved of parental oversight, qualitatively improve (Aquilino, 2006). A history of competent self-regulation, a childhood capacity with positive repercussions throughout development (Shonkoff & Phillips, 2000), predicts general improvements in family relationships.

Many critical choices loom in the minds of emerging adults. Parents' willingness to support their adult children is both helpful and infantilizing, removing reality pressure but promoting passivity. Nonetheless, career choice and financial independence have repercussions on family relationships and reverberate in interactions with friends and romantic partners. Feeling engaged in meaningful work makes the approach to an adult committed relationship seem more possible. This sequence has strong empirical support (Beyers & Seiffge-Krenke, 2010) and is frequently articulated in the clinical context. The problem is to define meaningful work, currently quite different from the past.

The prevalence of risk behaviors (associated with sensation-seeking thrills) and recklessness (associated with dangerous activities with little explicit peer approval) continues to rise in emerging adulthood, more so in men than women, but both men and women show the same trend. A study assessing overall reckless behavior in 18- to

29-year-olds shows that these behaviors steadily mount through college, graduation, and well into one's twenties. They tend to cluster together. For example, heavy episodic alcohol use during and after college is associated with other risk behaviors, including drunk driving, unprotected sex, and impulsive violence (Duangpatra, Bradley, & Glendon, 2009; Willoughby & Dworkin, 2008). Excessive alcohol use has been positively correlated with work intensity (Eitle et al., 2010). The association may reflect the working emerging adult's discretionary income and the reality that the entry-level work culture, like college culture (with the "college-effect" of incremental alcohol use [White & Jackson, 2004/2005]), promotes drinking. Modulating factors for risk behaviors are not plentiful: being married or expressing a conscious desire to be married are shown to consistently diminish alcohol consumption (Duncan, Wilkerson, & England, 2006), despite the finding that marriage has lost its status as an adult marker (Arnett, 2004). In addition, an orientation toward the future has been shown to have an overall moderating effect on recklessness (Duangpatra, Bradley, & Glendon, 2009). These findings suggest that consciousness of one's own imminent adulthood may be lagging well past its expected consolidation in the majority of emerging adults, and that psychotemporal adaptation, although cognitively possible, is stalled. Arnett's notion that these people continue to feel "in-between" (i.e., between childhood and adulthood) may be the best explanation available. In fact, the notion of adulthood is no longer described as an achievement. Terms such as "overwhelming," "the end of fun," and "stagnation" are offered to explain the dread of adulthood (Arnett, 2004, pp. 218–219). If traditionally defined adulthood, with all its requirements and obligations, is not a goal—because it is no longer revered, no longer contemporary, or no longer possible—then the psychological end of development stretches into a distant future.

Summary

Emerging adulthood, proposed as a new developmental phase by Jeffrey Arnett in 2000, has become the focus of hundreds of thousands of research studies. Variously placed between ages 18 to 24, 18 to 29, or 21 to 30, this phenomenon is somewhat obfuscated by its chronological and developmental boundaries, which blend into late adolescence.

Despite detractors in developmental science and longstanding controversy about adult development in psychoanalysis (see Abrams, 1990), Arnett's proposal has captured the interest of legions of developmental thinkers and identified a phenomenon that, however transient, is instantly recognizable to the media and the world at large. In our view, Arnett's description of emerging adulthood fits the 23- to 30-year-olds in contemporary society, a generation raised in the technocultural world. The impact of social media, relentless visual communication, and forced transparency must be considered, because these features of today's world will inevitably effect drastic changes in developmental experience.[7]

Today's emerging adults—recent college graduates, college dropouts, or high school graduates in the workforce for a few years—have all had a version of psychosocial moratorium post high school. Although full-time employed young men and women are more immersed in consequential reality than the average college student, most do not consider the job they have straight out of high school to be their real future. They still do not know what they are "going to be." At 23 or 24, both college graduates and their cohort in the workforce feel that their right to the (late adolescent) psychosocial moratorium has expired, but, to their dismay, they are unsure how to proceed in a world in which adulthood seems substantively different from what they observed in their parent's generation and how to get there remains obscure. They express uncertainty about direction, are less invested in achieving traditional adult commitments and responsibilities, and describe a subjective experience of suspension and ineffectiveness, unforeseen and unprecedented by prior generations. The relationship of their plight to the "postmodern condition" (or the post-postmodern condition) is a critical question, arguably too early to judge. These young people are in the grip of an extended identity dilemma, hopeful that they will find their way but lacking traditions or mentors to advise them in a radically changed world. Their suspension at the threshold depends upon their parents' partial or full financial support. Not infrequently this arrangement, which often involves returning to the parental home, aggravates their condition, heightening the feeling of being in-between and compromising the process of leveling the field that occurs between parents and their adult children. The phenomenon that Arnett astutely recognized and named may very well represent the first wave of young people whose mental lives and visions of the future reflect a fundamentally different kind of development, deeply shaped by early exposure to virtual reality, absence of privacy, changed family structures, and the hegemony of technology.

- Emerging adulthood is considered by many to be the new developmental phase of the twenty-first century. The literature is consistently inconsistent about the parameters of this cohort. In our view, the period from the early twenties to thirty encompasses the individuals who fit the description best.
- Jeffrey Arnett first characterized this cohort in 2000. His original description (which was of youth 18–24 years of age) identified five features: (1) Identity explorations; (2) instability; (3) heightened self-focus; (4) subjective feeling of being in-between; and (5) age of possibilities (Arnett, 2004, p. 8).
- There is considerable disagreement among developmental scholars about both development during adulthood and the concept of developmental phases. Psychoanalytic thinkers studying the adolescent process in the second half of the twentieth century (i.e., Erikson, Blos, and others), had already identified a post-adolescent consolidation or integration of personality, undoubtedly a part of what Arnett describes as the emerging adult experience. Identity formation is a visible manifestation, but the process is an intrapsychic one: full individuation, stabilization of patterned defenses and character, resolution of childhood

trauma, consolidation of sexual identity and object choice, and the establishment of ego continuity.

- Although there is growing evidence that brain development extends through the twenties, its relationship to the contemporary dilemma of emerging adults has not been clarified. Social factors of the twenty-first century, such as loss of traditional conduits to all the milestones of adulthood (i.e., marriage, career, childbearing), preeminence of technology and associated skills, globalization, changing attitudes toward cohabitation, and so on, play a part in this generation's particular burden.

- The developmental experience of children born after 1980 marks a significant departure from the past; today's millennials are the transitional generation grappling with adulthood in the technocultural era. As Western postindustrial society moves toward total immersion in digital culture, from infancy to old age, changes in mental life are inevitable. Social transformation of this magnitude and ubiquity will be reflected in the instinctual lives, relationships, values and morality, and personal integrity of generations to come.

Notes

1. The vast research literature on emerging adulthood spawned by Arnett's ideas is itself often ambiguous about the age group being considered, and the popular press has consistently favored a later time frame: They are "twenty-somethings" (Brooks, 2007; Henig, 2010) or 18- to 29-year-olds (Jayson, 2012).

2. Changes in the content of the superego due to the influence of peers, significant mentors, and/or the acquisition of power, wealth, or celebrity are well described in psychoanalytic literature (Arlow, 1982) and popular media (as in Dr. Robert Millman's description of "acquired situational narcissism" described in *The New York Times* [Sherrill, 2001].)

3. 40.5%, according to a *New York Times Business Day* April 28, 2010 article by Catherine Campbell.

4. Six years post–high school graduation, the rate of actual college graduates reported by the US Department of Education in 2012 ranged from 60.2% among white students to 37.9% among black students ("Breaking News," *Journal of Blacks in Higher Education*, October, 2012). In 2012, the US Census reported that 39.4% of all Americans between 25 and 34 have college degrees (reported in *Money Watch*, July 12, 2012).

5. A recent survey conducted by Harris interactive and published by Forbes (May 20, 2011) showed that 60% of parents support their young adult children after they finish school, providing an economic safety net that enables "wandering." However, because this younger generation's financial outlook is less favorable than their parents, they are unlikely to have means to offer a similar opportunity to their own children (Hendry & Kloep, 2007).

6. In his 2005 commencement address at Kenyon College, DFW began with this "didactic parable": There are these two young fish swimming along and they happen to meet an older fish swimming the other way, who nods at them and says, "Morning, boys. How's the water?" And the two young fish swim on for a bit, and then eventually one of them looks over at the other and goes "What the hell is water?"

7. *The Circle*, by Dave Eggars, takes a sardonic look at emerging adulthood on the fictional campus of a wrap-around, fast growing internet company, showing in harrowing, yet matter-of-fact detail the transformations wrought by the rules of the cyberworld: "Privacy is theft; secrets are lies."

References

Abrams, S. (1990). The psychoanalytic process: The developmental and the integrative. *Psychoanalytic Quarterly, 59*, 650–677.

Adatto, C. P. (1966). On the metamorphosis from sdolescence into adulthood. *Journal of the American Psychoanalytic Association, 14*, 485–509.

Aquilino, W. S. (2006). Family relationships and support systems in emerging adulthood. In J. J. Arnett & J. L. Tanner (Eds.), *Emerging*

Adults in America: Coming of Age in the 21st Century (pp. 193–217). Washington, DC: American Psychological Association.

Arlow, J. (1982). Problems of the superego concept. *Psychoanalytic Study of the Child, 37*, 229–244.

Arnett, J. J. (1997). Young people's conceptions of the transition to adulthood. *Youth & Society, 29*, 3–23.

Arnett, J. J. (2000). Emerging adulthood: a theory of development from the late teens through the twenties. *American Psychologist, 55*, 469–480.

Arnett, J. J. (2004). *Emerging Adulthood: The Winding Road from the Late Teens Through the Twenties*. Oxford, UK: Oxford University Press.

Arnett, J. J. (2005). The developmental context of substance use in emerging adulthood. *Journal of Drug Issues, 35*, 235–253.

Arnett, J. J. (2007). Suffering, selfish, slackers? Myths and reality about emerging adults. *Journal of Youth & Adolescence, 36*, 23–29.

Arnett, J. J., Kloep, M., Hendry L. B., & Tanner, J. L. (2011). *Debating Emerging Adulthood: Stage or Process?* Oxford, UK: Oxford University Press

Arnett, J. J. & Taber, S. (1994). Adolescence terminable and interminable: when does adolescence end? *Journal of Youth &Adolescence, 23*, 517–537.

Beck, M. (2012). Delayed development: 20-somethings blame the brain. *Health Journal of the Wall Street Journal*, August 23, 2012. http://online.wsj.com/news/articles/SB10000872396390443713704577601532208760746?mg=reno64wsj&url=http%3A%2F%2Fonline.wsj.com%2Farticle%2FSB10000872396390443713704577601532208760746.html

Beyers, W., & Seiffge-Krenke, I. (2010). Does identity precede intimacy? Testing Erikson's theory on romantic development in emerging adults of the 21st century. *Journal of Adolescent Research, 25*, 387–415.

Blakemore, S-J. (2012). Imaging brain development: the adolescent brain. *NeuroImage, 61*, 397–406.

Blos, P. (1954). Prolonged adolescence: the formulation of a syndrome and its therapeutic implications. *American Journal of Orthopsychiatry, 24*, 733–742.

Blos, P. (1962). *On Adolescence: A Psychoanalytic Interpretation*. New York: Free Press.

Blos, P. (1979). *The Adolescent Passage: Developmental Issues*. Madison, CT: International University Press.

Blum, H. P. (1985). Superego formation, adolescent transformation, and the adult neurosis. *Journal of the American Psychoanalytic Association, 33,* 887–909.

Brooks, D. (2007). The odyssey years. *New York Times Op-Ed,* December 7: http://www.nytimes.com/2007/10/09/opinion/09brooks.html

Bronk, K. C. (2011). A grounded theory of the development of noble youth purpose. *Journal of Adolescent Research, 27,* 78–109.

Bynner, J. (2005). Rethinking the youth phase of the life-course: the case for emerging adulthood? *Journal of Youth Studies, 8,* 367–384.

Colarusso, C. A. (1991). The development of time sense in young adulthood. *Psychoanalytic Study of the Child, 46,* 125–144.

Coupland, D. (1991). *Generation X: Tales for an Accelerated Culture.* New York: St. Martin's Press.

Duangpatra, K. N. K., Bradley, G. L., & Glendon, G. (2009). Variables affecting emerging adults' self-reported risk and reckless behaviors. *Journal of Applied Developmental Psychology, 30,* 298–309.

Duncan, G. J., Wilkerson, B., & England, P. (2006). Cleaning up their act: the effects of marriage and cohabitation on licit and illicit drug use. *Demography, 43,* 691–710.

Eggars, D. (2013). *The Circle.* New York: Knopf. In endnote

Eitle, D., Taylor, J., & Eitle T. M. (2010). Heavy episodic alcohol use in emerging adulthood: the role of early risk factors and young adult social roles. *Journal of Drug Issues, 20,* 295–320.

Erikson, E. H. (1956). The problem of ego identity. *Journal of the American Psychoanalytic Association, 4,* 56–121.

Erikson, E. H. (1970). Reflections on the dissent of contemporary youth. *International Journal of Psychoanalysis, 51,* 11–22.

Fabricius, J. (1998). Refusal of autonomy: the use of words by a young adult in analysis. *Journal of the Amercian Psychoanalytic Association, 46,* 105–120.

Furstenberg, F. F. (2010). On a new schedule: transitions to adulthood and family change. *The Future of Children, 20,* 67–87.

Hamilton, S. F., & Hamilton, M. A. (2006). School, work and emerging adulthood. In J. J. Arnett & J. L.Tanner (Eds.), *Emerging Adults in America: Coming of Age in the 21st Century* (pp. 257–277). Washington, DC: American Psychological Association.

Hall, G. S. (1904). *Adolescence: Its Psychology and Its Relations to Physiology, Anthropology, Sociology, Sex, Crime, Religion, and Education* (Vol I). New York: D. Appleton & Company.

Hendry, L. B. & Kloep, M. (2002). *Lifespan Development: Resources, Challenges and Risks*. London: Thomson Learning.

Hendry, L. B. & Kloep, M. (2007). Conceptualizing emerging adulthood: inspecting the emperor's new clothes? *Child Development Perspectives, 1,* 74–79.

Henig, R. M. (2010). What is it about 20-somethings? *New York Times Magazine,*August18,2010,http://www.nytimes.com/2010/08/22/magazine/22Adulthood-t.html?pagewanted=all&_r=0

Hu, E. (2013). This boardgame aims to teach preschoolers how to code. *NPR, All Tech Considered,* September 18, 2013, http://www.npr.org/blogs/alltechconsidered/2013/09/17/223402361/this-board-game-aims-to-teach-preschoolers-how-to-code

Jayson, S. (2012). Many "emerging adults" 18-29 are not there yet. *USA Today,* July 29, 2012, http://usatoday30.usatoday.com/news/health/wellness/story/2012-07-30/Emerging-adults-18-29-still-attached-to-parents/56575404/1

Keniston, K. (1968). *Young Radicals: Notes on Committed Youth.* New York: Harcourt Press.

Kernberg, O. (2006). Identity: recent findings and clinical implications. *Psychoanalytic Quarterly, 75,* 969–1003.

Konstam, V. (2007). *Emerging and Young Adulthood: Multiple Perspectives, Diverse Narratives.* New York: Springer-Verlag.

Laufer, M. (1978). The nature of adolescent pathology and the psychoanalytic process. *Psychoanalytic Study of the Child, 33,* 307–322.

Lebel, C. & Beaulieu, C. (2011). Longitudinal development of human brain wiring continues from childhood into adulthood. *Journal of Neuroscience, 31*(30), 10937–10947.

Marcia, J. (1993). The ego identity status approach to ego identity. In J. E. Marcia, A. S. Waterman, D. R. Matteson, S. I. Archer, & J. L. Orlofsky (Eds.), *Ego Identity: A Handbook of Psychosocial Research* (pp. 3–21). New York: Springer.

Sherrill, S. (2001). Acquired malignant narcissism. *The New York Times Magazine,* December 9 http://www.nytimes.com/2001/12/09/magazine/09ASN.html

Shonkoff, J. P., & Phillips, D. A. (2000). *From Neurons to Neighborhoods: The Science of Early Childhood Development.* Washington, DC: National Academy Press.

Tanner, J. (2006). Recentering during emerging adulthood: A critical turning point in life span human development. In J. Arnett & J. Tanner (Eds.), *Emerging Adults in America: Coming of Age in the 21st*

Century (pp. 21–55). Washington, DC: American Psychological Association.

Wallerstein, R. S. (1998). Erikson's concept of ego identity reconsidered. *Journal of the American Psychoanalytic Association, 46,* 229–247.

White, H. R. & Jackson, K. (2004/2005). Social and psychological influences on emerging adult drinking behavior. *Alcohol Research and Health, 28,* 182–190.

Willoughby, B. J. & Dworkin, J. (2008). The relationships between emerging adults' expressed desire to marry and frequency of participation in risk-taking behaviors. *Youth & Society, 40,* 426–450.

9

Conclusion: Why Study Development?

This description of human development from a psychoanalytic perspective is intended to foster awareness of how the human mind
evolves through a series of mental organizations, each with its own
cognitive and emotional capacities and each with its particular tasks
and achievements. Our belief is that such awareness can enhance
clinical sensitivity to the deeply interwoven past and present, ideally augmenting the clinician's contribution to the long and arduous
psychoanalytic process of self-discovery and creation of a coherent
sense of self—past, present, and future. Knowledge of "possible
developmental paths" (P. Tyson, 1998, p. 12) and sequential mental
organizations that characterize children's minds over the course of
childhood and adolescence deepens clinical work with adults in the
following ways:

First, it facilitates recognition of transference paradigms, alerting the clinician to "old patterns of interacting with others, old patterns of resolving conflict ... (that) creep gradually into the analytic
process despite the opportunities it offers for change" (P. Tyson,
1998, p. 12). In this we endorse the notion that the individual entering the analytic relationship brings his or her own set of screen
memories, unconscious fantasies, characteristic coping strategies,
and object relational expectations and patterns to the analytic relationship. Of course, the analyst has a similar set of idiosyncratic
intrapsychic components, presumably understood via a training
analysis, well enough to allow the gradual clarification of what factors belong predominately to the patient, the analyst and/or their
synergy.

Second, such knowledge transforms what every analyst already possesses—his or her developmental "theory fragments, almost-theories, and pseudotheories" (Gopnik, 1996, p. 221)—into a better informed, realistic, enlightened, and realized picture of development. Developmental theories are a fundamental part of everyone's mental life (Gilmore, 2008; Mayes, 1999), present in fantasy, attitudes, hopes, relationships, educational endeavors, and so on. They inform our notions of how humans grow and change, thereby entering into our approaches to a host of activities: teaching, learning, the endless choices made raising children, arguing with family members, negotiating, and so on. Such theories are sanctuaries for prejudicial ideas (for example, about race, women, homosexuality, to name a few) and antiquated notions, even old wives' tales (such as, only-children are shy, spoiled, aggressive, and/or maladjusted [Newman, 2001/1990] or that there is a nonverbal period of development [Vivona, 2012]). While these can be maintained in our personal lives, they have no place in our clinical work.

As child clinicians, it seems self-evident that our capacity to comprehend our patients' narratives depends on understanding how the mind develops and how such narratives are created, but this conviction is nonetheless difficult to document. Psychoanalytic training introduces candidates to the psychoanalytic baby of their institute's theoretical school, and so every analyst emerges from his or her education informed by conceptions of development gleaned from that baby and myriad other sources, from curricular to personal. The more those conceptions are tempered by knowledge of developmental paradigms and plots that are actually possible, the more we can understand the layers of childhood fantasy, cognition, defense, and environmental provision in our patients. We are all in danger of forcing a patient's story into our own notions of how development happens (Cooper, 1989); it is far better to ground our clinical work in our knowledge of the realities of developmental progression.

Of course, the same caution applies to the approach we describe throughout this book: Modern ego psychology has its own emphasis and perspective and our very insistence on the importance of developmental knowledge reflects it Because we believe that the integration of advances in understanding the developing mind are crucial to preserving psychoanalysis as a vital discipline, we have shaped this introductory volume by interfacing with contemporary developmental science and strongly endorse receptivity to new findings to come. We are aware of postmodern philosophical objections to positivist empiricism and recognize that "knowledge" is highly dependent on cultural context and perspective. However, at this moment, in this culture, we can make use of information as it applies to development here and now. In this regard, it seems ironic that many postmodern schools that disclaim interest in development actually arose out of infant observation (Cooper, 1989) and contemporary developmental neuroscience. The many related disciplines that investigate human development are a rich, continuous source of psychoanalytic innovation (Cooper, 1989; Govrin, 2006; Vivona, 2012).

We believe that knowing how the mind develops illuminates work with each individual patient in every clinical encounter. Knowledge of prior modalities of functioning are crucial to making sense of patient's communications, which can fluctuate because of shifts in ego state over the course of a single session (Dowling, 2004). Maximal interpretive mileage from exploration of screen memories depends on understanding the mind that registered them (Lafarge, 2012) and their current purpose (Reichbart, 2008). Despite declining interest, screen memories are invaluable portals to our patient's inner lives and histories as well as their self-representations, in the past and the present. Similarly, unconscious fantasy is best understood by knowing the naïve cognition and wishful thinking of childhood that shaped perception, deepening comprehension of the parameters and constraints that operated at time of its emergence and its evocation and transformation at different points in development (Erreich, 2003). In general, the patient's anamnesis is inevitably, mostly unconsciously, evaluated in the course of analysis in terms of what we believe is developmentally possible. The more we know of developmental constellations, infant capacities, and the developmental realities of our society, the better we can hear the interplay of defense, fantasy, and subjective experience in our patient's narrative (Cooper, 1989).

As we proposed elsewhere (Gilmore & Meersand, 2013), knowledge of development is like a good guidebook to an interesting, complex city with a unique history and evolution. We learn our way around it by appreciating the changing configurations and purposes of its neighborhoods over time—the shifting location of its administrative center, landmarks and their meanings, areas of poverty and gentrification, waves of immigrants and their introduction of foreign cultures, and the residue of catastrophic events and their solutions, both natural and man-made. To be of value to the current visitor, such a guidebook must be continuously updated by new historical discoveries and new interpretations of old ones— of excavated ancient sites, anthropological researches, and theoretical reconsiderations of its past—and by inclusion of current demographics, urban development projects, crime patterns, and transformations of old structures for new uses. Just as an old guidebook will provide no insight into contemporary rehabilitations and changes of purpose, recent transformations of boundaries and ethnic concentrations, contractions resulting from changes in economy, or current thinking about the historical organizations and reorganizations of the city, so too our developmental guidebook will fail us if it is not revised and updated, not only by a deeper understanding of the patient, but also by incorporating new knowledge about development.

We share the developmental scientists' conviction that there is no unitary developmental theory; development is too complicated, multisystemic, serendipitous, and extravagant to permit a single explanatory theory. This book is an exercise in selecting theories that fit our observations, understanding that our observations are colored by our general orientation toward psychoanalytic thinking as interpreted by modern ego psychology and the culture at large. We hope that we have adequately acknowledged our debt to the many ideas outside that domain that contribute to our understanding of our patients and that we have provided the reader with an approach that is enlightened, flexible, and open-minded.

References

Cooper, A. (1989). Infant research and adult psychoanalysis. In S. Dowling & A. Rothstein (Eds.), *The Significance of Infant Observational Research for Clinical Work with Children, Adolescents, and Adults* (pp. 79–89). Workshop Series of the American Psychoanalytic Association, Monograph 5. Madison, CT: International Universities Press.

Dowling, S. (2004). A reconsideration of the concept of regression. *Psychoanalytic Study of the Child, 58,* 191–210.

Erreich, A. (2003). A modest proposal: (re)defining unconscious fantasy. *Psychoanalytic Quarterly, 72,* 541–574.

Gilmore, K. (2008). Psychoanalytic developmental theory: a contemporary reconsideration. *Journal of the American Psychoanalytic Association, 56,* 885–907.

Gilmore, K. & Meersand, P. (2013). *Normal child and adolescent development: a psychodynamic primer.* Washington, DC: American Psychiatric Publishing.

Gopnik, A. (1996). The post-Piaget era. *Psychological Science, 7,* 221–225.

Govrin, A. (2006). The dilemma of contemporary psychoanalysis: toward a "knowing" post post-modernism. *Journal of the American Psychoanalytic Association, 54,* 507–535.

Lafarge, L. (2012). The screen memory and the act of remembering. *International Journal of Psychoanalysis, 93,*1249–1265.

Mayes, L. C. (1999). Clocks, engines, and quarks—love, dreams, and genes: what makes development happen? *Psychoanalytic Study of the Child, 54,* 169–192.

Newman, S. (2001/1990). *Parenting an Only Child: The Joys and Challenges of Raising Your One and Only.* New York: Broadway Books.

Reichbart, R. (2008). Screen memory: its importance to object relations and transference. *Journal of the American Psychoanalytic Association, 56,* 455–481.

Tyson, P. (1998). Developmental theory and the postmodern psycho-analyst. *Journal of the American Psychoanalytic Association, 46,* 9–15.

Vivona, J. M. (2012). Is there a nonverbal period of development? *Journal of the American Psychoanalytic Association, 60,* 231–265.

Glossary

Component identities: The multiple identities, such as sexual orientation, race, gender, and religion, that figure in the determination of sociocultural power and privilege. Intersectionality theory originated in women's studies to refer to how components, such as race and gender, intersect and interlock, to create their own meanings.

Concrete operations: A period of cognitive development, between ages 7 and 11, in which children acquire the capacity for logical mental actions (operations). Thought is increasingly available as trial action. Children are able to maintain internal principles such as conservation and reversibility when faced with apparent changes in the appearance of an object.

Decentration: A hallmark of the concrete operational period, this capacity allows children to detach their thinking from an egocentric, perceptually bound perspective and consider multiple viewpoints.

Ego ideal: Currently defined in *Psychoanalytic Terms and Concepts* (2012) as a component of the superego that maintains standards, values, and ideals. Some theorists, such as Blos, consider it the residue of the negative oedipal complex, an internalization of the idealized features of the same sex object that supports an idealized self-representation.

Executive functions: An integrative set of mental functions that guides goal-directed actions and personal behavior, including such cognitive controls as shifting attention, planning, and voluntary inhibition of responses.

Externalization: A typical latency-phase defensive process in which children solicit environmental conflict and punishment in order to avoid the discomfort of internal guilt and superego conflicts.

Formal operations: Piaget described this cognitive period of development, which emerges in early adolescence, as characterized by capacities for hypothetical-deductive reasoning and higher level abstraction.

Identity diffusion: Used normatively by Erikson and in Marcia's research, this term designates a period of exploration or noncommitment that is on the way to identity achievement. However, it has come to be associated with borderline personality disorder in Kernberg's writings. For Kernberg (2006), identity diffusion reflects the sustained presence of multiple, contradictory self- representations that lack cohesiveness and contribute to the subjective feeling of emptiness.

Identity status: Marcia (1993) operationalized Erikson's concepts to assess "identity status." He observed four "types": diffusion (low commitment, exploration, and conflict), foreclosure (low exploration due to acceptance of parental values and expectations), moratorium (high exploration and low commitment), and achievement (high exploration and commitment). These types can evolve over time, with most youth moving toward achievement.

Libidinal object constancy: The capacity to maintain a unified, stable internalized representation of relationships despite transient or situational stressors.

Mentalization: Emerging at around the age of four years, mentalization is the capacity to grasp mental states. It is closely linked to the quality of parent–child attachment and emotional sharing, and to the child's affective sense of self.

Millennials: The generation coming of age in the first decades of the twenty-first century. In comparison with prior generations, they are more likely to have been raised in a single-parent home, more invested in social media for access to the peer group, more focused on visual imagery and instant communication, and more liberal-minded and confident (Pew Research Center).

Nonlinear systems theory: The dominant scientific paradigm of the twentieth century that focuses on the organization of the whole, rather than the parts. Simple explanations of etiology are replaced by the notion of temporary states achieved by a vast array of involved systems. Informed by modern mathematical advances that have revealed general laws of systems, nonlinear systems theory has been applied to the gamut of scientific endeavors, describing transformation through multiple interacting, evolving, and contributing systems. Human development as a whole and any facet of development should be examined as the product of multiple processes, themselves in evolution.

Object removal: The process by which adolescents, under pressure from increased sexual and aggressive urges, turn decisively away from their parental (oedipal) relationships toward other objects, usually amongst their peers.

Preoperational thinking: A period of cognitive development, beginning at about 18 months, in which semiotic functions emerge. The toddler manifests deferred imitation, acquires both language and early forms of play, and begins to apply mental rather than sensorimotor processes to solving problems.

Primal scene: A paradigm of erotic arousal and accompanying feelings of painful exclusion. This term is sometimes used to refer concretely to the child's witnessing of parental sexual activity.

Prolonged adolescence: A term coined by Peter Blos originally to designate young men who faltered when faced with the requirements that they resolve the adolescent crisis, individuate, and apply themselves to preparation for a realistic future. For these young men, inflated and sustained by parental narcissism that bore no relationship to their efforts, "their great future lies behind them" (Blos, 1954, p. 737).

Psychic equivalence: A mode of thinking in which very young children equate inner thoughts and feelings with reality.

Psychosocial moratorium: The term coined by Erikson (1965) to designate the interim offered in Western cultures for the late adolescent's identity exploration. Institutionalized in the college experience, the moratorium allowed youth to experiment with roles in order to establish self-sameness and continuity that are recognized by society.

Rapprochement: A phase of toddler development, beginning at about 15 to 18 months of age, wherein the child's increased awareness of self and separateness creates renewed separation anxieties and intensified wishes for maternal contact.

Second individuation: Blos derives this term from Mahler's separation-individuation theory, using it to illustrate the dramatic reduction in the adolescent's intimacy and dependency vis-à-vis the parents.

Technoculture: The ascendance of information technology and its impact on how culture is transmitted from generation to generation. The rise of the internet has altered many aspects of development, some not yet realized. Examples include the evolution of peer relationships, conceptualizations of reality, access to the forbidden, preponderance of the visual, foundations of "knowing," and cultural values.

The family romance: This universal latency fantasy, which involves imagining a special and powerful birthright (e.g., royal or magical parents) that has been lost, serves to assuage the school-aged child's increasing need to confront reality, particularly diminished idealization of the parents and the knowledge of personal limitations.

The wished-for self-image: In Milrod's elaboration of object relations theory, this applies to a substructure within the ego that represents admired qualities and behaviors (usually derived from the parents) for which the toddler strives, often manifested via imitation of parental actions.

Theory of mind: A network of concepts, demonstrable by around age four years, which govern how people predict and interpret others' behaviors, including the realization that beliefs (even when false) drive people's actions. It is related to mentalization, but theory of mind is generally considered a more cognitively based notion.

Traditional schools: Those identified as Freudian, ego psychological, Kleinian, and neo-Kleinian, Bionian, Winnicottian, Jungian, and self-psychological. *Postmodern* or *post postmodern* refers to the relational, interpersonal, co-constructionist, and intersubjective schools.

Youth culture: A term arising in the 1950s to describe the way adolescents set themselves apart from the adult generation. Although likely true throughout human history, the term arose with the growing interval between puberty and adulthood to highlight the different fads, slang, music, and lifestyle values that characterize the younger generation.

Index